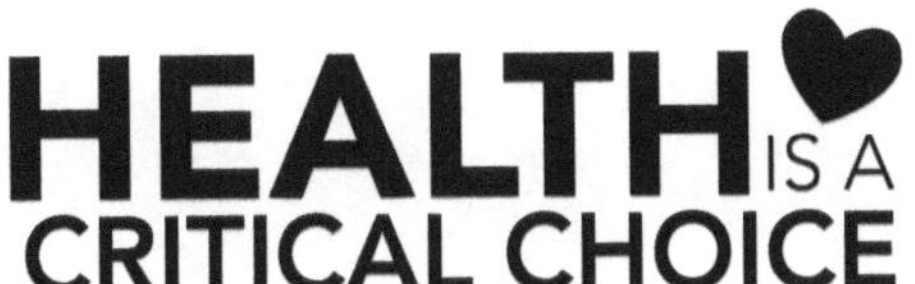
HEALTH IS A
CRITICAL CHOICE

HEALTH 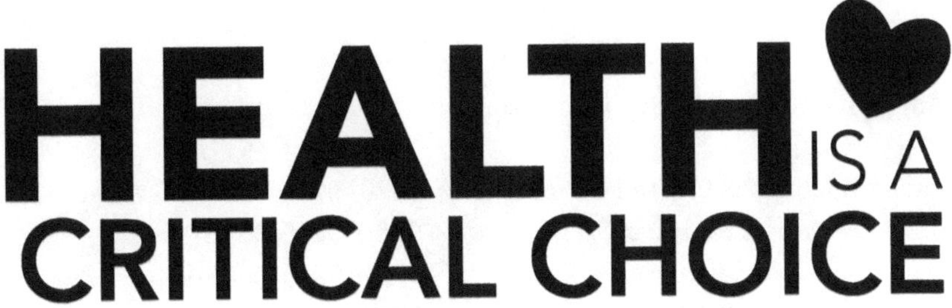 IS A CRITICAL CHOICE

Choose to Live Healthier, Happier and Longer

ALICK JAMES BANDA

To order additional copies of this book, contact:
Xlibris
1-800-455-039
www.Xlibris.com.au
Orders@Xlibris.com.au
812952

CONTENTS

DISCLAIMER

This book does not contain or intend to give medical advice, but it is meant for educational and informational purposes only. The book is not projected to replace professional medical advice, diagnosis, prognosis or treatment. Kindly consult your medical doctor for personalised medical advice and always seek out the advice of a physician or other qualified healthcare providers with any questions regarding a medical condition. Never neglect or defer seeking specialised medical guidance or treatment because of something you read in this book.

INTRODUCTION

It is estimated that every 52 seconds, someone dies of a chronic ailment like stroke or heart disease. About 60% of the more than 50 million total reported deaths in the world, are said to be associated with chronic illness. Almost half of them are attributed to cardiovascular diseases. That picture looks bleak! But the good news is that an estimated over 80% of those non-communicable diseases like diabetes, obesity, high blood pressure, stroke, coronary artery disease and cancer can be prevented as well as possibly reversed. Current studies show that genetics is only a smaller percent of the health equation, because lifestyle and nutrition remain high on the scale with toxins, stress, sedentary life and excess medication contributing to deadly health outcomes.

Have you ever woken up feeling so tired or indeed that you should not get out of bed? Have you ever felt like your body is not yours, lacking the energy that you so deserve? Have you ever felt so stressed, depressed, anxious, fatigued and brain fogged? If you answered *yes* to any of those questions, well, several of us have felt like that before. So, you are not alone. That feeling could be caused by a number of factors, but chief among them, is certainly what you eat and what you do with what you eat.

We are not supposed to get sick, but most times, we choose to get sick or feel bad due to what we put in us and our lifestyle. There is no known or convincing justification why we should have non-communicable illnesses of diabetes, cancer, obesity, high blood pressure, heart disease and stroke among others. Diseases are not supposed to predetermine how fast we grow old, but we have the fortitude and tenacity not to get ill.

In the year 2000, I bought a book called *"Where There Is No Doctor: A Village Healthcare Handbook."* The Book is a manual published by Hesperian Health Guides, with authors David Werner, Carol Thuman and Jane Maxwel from the United States of America. It is based on the experiences of David Werner at his Project Piaxtla, western Mexico. It was originally written in 1970 in Spanish as *Donde No Hay Doctor*. It tackles virtually all facets of the health of the people, such as malaria, bone fractures, ringworms and diarrhoea among others. Particular stress is put on cleanliness, vaccinations and a diet that's healthy. The book spells what people *can personally do* and how to avoid, distinguish and take care of many illnesses that are frequent. It also illustrates how to pinpoint difficulties they are incapable to deal with and referring to a health care authority...

But for me at that time, I kept wondering why such a book was written and *why shouldn't there be a doctor and why should there be?* I kept asking myself. But as I read through it, that's when it downed on me that there are many things that we can do without a doctor to keep healthy because doctors are not entirely the answer to our health; *we hold the key to our health*. The notion that when I go to the hospital and see a doctor is the only way to get better, has been engulfed in our entire lives and that is why we think we cannot do anything ourselves to stay healthy without a doctor. Do not get me wrong! Doctors are wonderful and helpful professionals, because they do so much and attend to our various emergency cases, anatomy, physiology, diagnosis, prognosis and medication among many important health matters. We need them as acute as it gets.

But let us face it; physicians can only do so much and food, nutrition and lifestyle, seem not to be part of most of their equation or agenda. They spend little time with patients (on average 5 minutes) and nutrition is not a hurry-hurry matter! Unfortunately, chronic illnesses that are currently killing us in millions, border on what you and I eat and our lifestyle. It is imperative to address a nutrition and lifestyle matter with a nutrition and lifestyle solution, rather than to administer a drug or medication as a solution. Our bodies are continuously telling us what they need and more often than not, we ignore their inaudible signals, until it is too late to listen and the body is now shouting out loudly. And instantly, we want the doctor to calm the shouts.

To live happier, healthier and longer, we should choose good health regarding the nutrition we have and the lifestyle we lead. Our bodies are self-regulating and restoring, but only if we support them with the right conditions. Advanced modern drugs and equipment, radiation, hospital operations are not very effective because all they do is subdue the signs and symptoms, unlike addressing the root cause of the ailment. Most of the drugs were crafted (intentionally or not) to address infectious diseases and this has worked to a large extent. But the current scourge is on the non-infectious illnesses, which are escalating at an alarming rate unabated.

Sickness comes about due to the body's lack of equilibrium over prolonged periods of time. But it is never too late to change your food, nutrition and lifestyle for the better, because you hold the power and key to that choice.

Let me make it clear from the beginning. *I am no doctor at all.* I am an advocate of a *Whole Food Plant-Based Nutrition*, because I have read, seen and experienced the amazing results that come with it. It was also because of the interest I developed in this kind of food, that I decided to become a Health and Wellness Life Coach and undertook some courses in healthcare, diet and nutrition and write books about it. And so, am proud and happy to promote this kind of food and lifestyle because it may just save the life of one or two people. Ultimately, we need healthy communities and nations where its people live healthier, happier and longer lives, while remaining useful and productive.

Raymond Francis, in his book, *The Great American Health Hoax*, talks about the confusing classification of over 12,000 different diseases in the world. But he says there is only one disease: *Malfunctioning Cells*. He notes that this is so because a cell is a microscopic unit of life where each one of us started from and this cell grew into trillions of cells to make tissues, organs and ultimately our bodies. Because cells are what make life possible, therefore, we need to understand what our cells need and what would cause them not to work well. Once the cell has what it needs and once it is not given what it does not need, then health is guaranteed. Therefore, the cause of disease is *Malfunctioning Cells*, and this comes about due to *toxicity* and *deficiency*. Raymond says if you are sick, it means you are not treating your cells accordingly and that by the time you get that ill, it means a lot of your cells are actually highly malfunctioning.

I do agree with Raymond, because if things are simplified in that way, it will be easier for anyone to underscore that I need to give my cells what they want and not poisons. If I do that, I won't be sick unnecessarily. We should not take disease as something that is normal, that should happen to us anytime and waiting for it to take place anyway! I remember a colleague of mine telling me about a friend who was diagnosed with diabetes. In telling me more details about it he said, *"You know these diseases, we live with them, it's part of life!"* I asked him "What?" It is not! We, indeed, like to give the responsibility for our health to someone else as well as blaming others: the doctor, the environment, the water and so on. Health is an important choice and it is our own full responsibility.

No one is 100% healthy and we are all going to die one day, but while we are still alive, it should be desirable that we live just a little bit healthier, longer, happier, well and fit. There is no one responsible for your health, not even your doctor or nurse. You are. I wrote this book for you. It is for you to ponder on the choices you make about your food and lifestyle. The fact that you are reading this book right now, means you do give a damn about your health and congratulations! What you are about to read here might change your life for better. You can live without being sick. The choice is simply yours.

MY EXPERIENCE

In 2013, I suffered from perpetual stomach upset problems. Whatever I ate, would cause me a lot of stomach rumbling, intermittent pain and diarrhoea. When I could not bear it anymore, I decided to go to the hospital. After some diagnostic tests at one of the renowned private hospitals in Chelstone, Lusaka, Zambia, the doctor prescribed for me about 15 medications. Okay, maybe you didn't get that right, FIFTEEEN, was the number of drugs given to me. With their courtesy and because of the huge number of medicine, they even gave me a plastic bag to carry those medicines in. When I looked at the medicines, I asked myself: *Surely, am I that sick, and that bad*? And where will all this medicine go? In my body? Because doctors emphasise that for the drugs to be effective, you MUST finish the course even if you feel better. If you stop taking the medication midway, (antibiotics for instance), the bacteria might not be gotten rid of, as required and when someone gets ill again, the bacteria that's outstanding, becomes antibiotic resistant.

Fast forward in February 2017, while in Canberra, Australia and serving as Zambia's diplomat to that country, I one day felt some bulging thing near my right breast. This didn't feel comfortable at all! Despite it being not painful, I could feel its presence and kept wondering what it was. I finally decided to go and see the General Practitioner at Philip Medical Centre in Woden. The doctor recommended that they do tests on me such as a biopsy, blood test and others. Four days later, I went back to see the GP. I was told that the *"thing"* was not suspected cancerous, but a possible lymph node in which some fat could have accumulated after possible injury. He further told me that I should *not worry* because it was not life threatening and may subside on its own. Did you hear me? The doctor said *I should not worry.* Come on! For over 40 years of my life, I have had no such a bulging thing on my body and then now lo and behold, am told I should not worry! Really? I thought I had all the rights to worry, because anything strange on my body calls for worry and concern, especially in this time and age of chronic illnesses, cancer among the deadliest. Though not very clear, the results of the tests are shown in the report below:

Phillip Diagnostic Imaging

Patient: Alick Banda
Subject: Us Breast (S) (R)
Result Date: 03/02/2017 00:00

Radiology Report:
Right Breast Ultrasound

Lump corresponds to well defined area of low density, measuring 16.0mm in the deep subcutaneous tissues overlying the pectoral muscles. There is internal density, which may represent internal fat. There is no cystic or calcific degeneration and the lesion is not thought to represent a cyst.

Conclusion

There is an unusual rounded lesion with a central area of possible fat. This may represent an unusual lymph node or possibly, a complex cyst with internal echoes but other soft tissue lesions cannot be excluded and I recommend an ultrasound guided aspirate or biopsy for further assessment in this patient if appropriate. The features are thought unlikely to represent sinister pathology…

A few months later, I went home, to Lusaka, Zambia. The *thing* on my breast was still bothering me and I decided to see another doctor for a possible second or third opinion. At the hospital, I was told that I needed to schedule an appointment for a scan and maybe an x-ray. Due to pressure of work, because I was busy checking on some of my construction projects, I did not make that appointment. I, therefore, decided to see my long-time friend doctor, Dr. K. Imasiku. The first thing I was told by Dr. Imasiku was that the lump was not a serious ailment because *there were people who were suffering from serious issues and not what I had,* but the doctor still recommended that if I wanted it removed, I could still go ahead and see one of the other doctors at some clinic within Lusaka. Two days later, I went to see the other doctors, male and female. Both of them were equally not sure what the *thing* was, but were also quick to hint that it might not be that serious and the best would be for me to ignore it or if I insisted, I should make an appointment to have it removed through a 'small surgery". I never made that appointment and two weeks later, I went back to Australia.

A year later, I had just subscribed to *Netflix Australia* and it seemed very exciting with a number of movies and documentaries. But one documentary that caught my eye was called *What the Health*, a film about diet and disease and the billions of dollars being spent on healthcare. Then I flipped on and watched *Fat Sick and Nearly Dead (1&2)* by an Australian, *Joe Cross* in which he talked about juicing and healing and his co-star Phill, a once obese guy. Then I watched *Folks Over Knives*, a film about the popularity of processed foods leading to obesity and other chronic illnesses. And I watched another film, *In Defense of Food* by Prof. Michael Pollan and yet another one called *That*

Sugar Film and other YouTube documentaries on *Whole Food Plant Based Diet*. I was overwhelmed. It got me to seriously start thinking about what I put in my body. I started imagining why we spend so much time and so much money on sicknesses that the body itself can attend to through what we feed it.

*　　*　　*

I love playing soccer, what others call social football. In Canberra, Australia Capital Territory, we used to play this social football at a place called O'Connor Playing Fields, in Turner, Pedder Street, off MacArthur Avenue, every Sunday afternoon till late evening. One Sunday afternoon in February 2019, we were as usual playing and one of my colleagues hit me with his elbow at my left rib cage. It really pained and I had to excuse myself, because I could not play properly.

I went home and tried to massage the area and applied some rub- on to try and ease the pain. The following morning, as I went for work, I could still feel excruciating pain. I used to use public transport most times to and from work. Two days later, as I walked from the bus station to my house, I could not manage to walk on a steep road because the pain at my rib cage was unbearable. When I arrived home, I was in deep pain and lay on the bed head down. I had to rush to the hospital to see the GP. The GP diagnosed me and told me that sports injuries were not supposed to take long to heal, which means I was badly injured because the pain had persisted. He then recommended that I do a Magnetic Resonance Imaging (MRI) and/or a Computer Tomography (CT) Scan to ascertain the gravity of the problem. I was advised to make an appointment with the department within the hospital that offered that service. I did make the appointment for the following day.

But when I went home, I had a second thought over the scan. Reading a book by Raymond Francis on *"Never Be Sick Again"* on the dangers of most drugs, certain radiations, rays and electromagnetic waves and how adverse these affect our cells, I got thinking about what the best way for me could be. I therefore decided to let it be and see how it may heal itself naturally using the body's amazing mechanisms and the food that I would be eating. So, I did not go for the scan.

How did I feel after?

Let me tell you the last part of my experience, but I will start with my father, after embarking on whole foods plant-based nutrition. My dad, James Chawinga Banda, was diagnosed with prostate cancer in 2015. It had reached an advanced stage and by the time we were taking him to the University Teaching Hospital (UTH) in Lusaka, Zambia, he was in a bad state. At 73, he, however, managed to undergo successful surgeries but, he was strongly advised to embark on a whole foods plant-based diet and avoid processed food as much as possible.

My dad has always been a disciplinarian and we grew up in such a disciplined environment all our lives. What I didn't know was that he was equally very disciplined to follow what the health personnel told him at the hospital. And so, he followed what he was told: no red meat, no sugar, no white flour products, no salt, no cooking oil and no milk. among others.

He decided to follow that and indeed concentrated on eating more plant-based food, *religiously*. The results, he told me, *were amazing and phenomenal.* He no longer had backaches, he no longer had elevated and frequent high blood pressures, no migraines and what not. He was fairly in good health, albeit his age. When at one time he went for review at UTH, the doctors told him that they were unable to exactly see the prostate cancer cells. That is what plant-based nutrition could do.

*   *   *

After watching all those documentaries, I told you initially and getting busy to read several nutrition and health books and doing several nutrition and diet courses, I also decided to try the lifestyle. From the day I made that decision, in 2017, instantly and first and foremost, I dropped sugar, whether white or brown. That was gone. I did away with all fizzy drinks or soft drinks. I did away with milk and tremendously reduced many dairy products except a few chunks of cheese. I also reduced on oil, especially vegetable oils, (other than taking some extra virgin olive oil that's cold pressed, sparingly). I started eating more cruciferous vegetables: broccoli, cauliflower, kale, cabbage and others. I was taking beans nearly every day; fruits, especially oranges, watermelons, apples, bananas and kiwi fruits were a daily treat. I would eat at least three fruits a day and a serving or two of vegetables or salads. Sometimes my breakfast would just comprise fruits and peanuts. Later at lunch I would have a bowl of salads, followed an hour later with green or white tea. During super, I would have some lump of starch carbohydrate from corn meal with plenty of pink cabbage or kale and beans. I would still eat some salmon and sardines sparsely. I would eat organic chicken once in a week and organic meat once in two or three weeks.

You certainly want to know the outcome of my above choices. My weight got a diving nose. I was weighing 72Kgs and just after two months, I lost 10 Kgs and that has been maintained steadily, notwithstanding issues of adjusting the sizes of my clothes. My stomach problems were all gone and I never felt a single pain or diarrhoea once I ate any food. The *thing* that was growing on my shoulder equally died a natural death or indeed got into some disappearing act. I could no longer feel it on my left shoulder area. The sports injury I suffered was also gone in an unknown circumstance, but surely because of the food I was eating. My skin changed for the better: it was softer and looked appealing, to me at least. My energy had been amazing! I felt no fatigue when waking up in the morning and never felt like sleeping on when it was time to wake up. I still played soccer and sprinted a lot and generally exercise like a 20-year-old boy. My friend Wiza Phiri even commented that *I was now aging backwards.*

HIGHLY PROCESSED OR REFINED FOOD

I guess you know and recall that processed food tastes nice, delicious and sumptuous. It is so appealing, and we just want to have a little more and more. Why?

Processed food, refined food or discretionary food, or food with *discovered nutrients (Dr. Joel Fuhrman, Super Immunity, 2011)*, is categorised as food which has extremely been treated and most often stripped of its original nutrient content, especially fibre. It can also be viewed as any deliberate modification in a food that occurs before it is available for consumption. Note that cooking, drying or freezing of food can also be looked at as a modest way of processing, to preserve nutrients and freshness. The catch word here is *modest*. When the *modest* is disregarded or ignored, we get to *highly processed*, especially with the aim of maintaining longer shelf life of the processed food.

Highly refined or processed food is produced in massive volumes and is uniform in its packaging. It is also found in the same manner in all countries one can go to with use of unique or precise ingredients. This food can be found almost everywhere you go like in supermarkets, convenience stores at gas or filling stations, fast food eating places, vending machines and so on. The food usually has extended shelf life which is one of the main focus of the food industry, as this culminates into the commodification of the food. At the end of the day, food is merely treated as a commodity without consideration of the value it must have to the buyer and his or her health. The ultimate goal is to make money and not think of health.

Some examples of highly refined or processed foods include table sugar, white flour, pasta, cheese, tinned vegetables, white bread, snacks (such as sausage rolls, pasties, pies), meat products (like sausage, bacon, salami, ham), cakes, biscuits, carbonated drinks, sweetened milk, pizza and so on.

It is important to underscore that not all food that is processed is deemed bad. There are certain foods that need to be processed to be safe for human consumption. An example would be milk which requires to be pasteurised to rid it of harmful bacteria. Most mushroom also has to be cooked, just like beans. Some food will not be used if it is not processed, like the need to process seeds to yield oil. Cooking may also be necessary to expose more enzymes of the food as well as make it palatable, such as cooking beans and some meats. Research shows that once tomato is cooked or made into paste, the antioxidant Lycopene in it, is more bioavailable. *(A Carotenoid, Lycopene is a pigment that's natural, giving fruits and vegetables the colour red. As an antioxidant, it safeguards damage of cells. Red Carrots, Guavas, Papayas and Watermelons, all are known to harbour Lycopene).*

So, it is therefore important to take note that food would be considered harmful because of it being *highly* processed and the element of additives such as sugar, salt and trans-fat, which are added to enhance flavour and be more attractive and improve its shelf life. For example, Mono Sodium Glutamate (MSG) is a food enhancer, that adds flavour to the food. It intensifies the meaty, savoury flavour, just like glutamate that occurs in nature will do in stews and meat soups. The MSG, however, is thought of having an effect of causing human beings to return for more food which booms the food industry but makes an individual vulnerable to disease. Human beings and animals are known to have reflex actions that tell them *to eat and to stop eating* after having enough. But with additives like MSG, and others, scientists state that it makes human beings keep eating because the food keeps tasting good, in the midst of long-term adverse effects. It is argued that more than 4000 supermarkets have products that contain MSG, as a known food additive.

In this regard, purchasing such kind of highly refined food may result in people taking too much of that particular food because of the enhanced flavour that makes them eat more. Equally, you may eat too much sugar or salt beyond the recommended amounts because you are not cognisant of how much was added to the food you bought and ate. It is possible that such foods might also be high in calories because of the high levels of fat and sugar. Subsequently, the sugars (glucose) from the refined or processed foods are gradually released into the person's bloodstream. For instance, eating slices of white bread, is such that the food industry makes the wheat used to make bread, undergo a process in which the bran and fibre, that is nourishing to the body, almost absent by the time we buy bread from the supermarket.

Dr. Robert Lustig, who is a Paediatrician and long-time childhood-obesity expert at California University, San Francisco, indicated that processed foods have affected Americans by increased intake of processed carbohydrates, increased Type 2 diabetes, obesity, environmental harm and spending more on health care.

Facets of Processed Food

Excess Sugar

Almost all of the highly processed food has high levels of sugar, particularly fructose. High Glycaemic Index, (GI), food (*which is a number indicating the comparative capability of a food, especially a carbohydrate, to boost the blood glucose level*), such as table sugar, sweets and some chocolates, increases blood sugar faster than food with a lower GI. Food with high amounts of sugar rapidly spike glucose and insulin levels, that cause increased androgen secretion and inflammation, all of which play a critical role in chronic illness. Sugar is a disaccharide containing monosaccharaides of glucose and fructose. It is fructose that is broken down in the liver and causes havoc once excesses are recorded. This would register problems like fatty liver and liver cirrhosis over time.

Studies show that sugar overstimulates reward centres and that brings about addiction because these centres of the brain are activated. Additionally, a big volume of dopamine hormone is released, that enables taking of sugar feel so nice, because dopamine is a hormone in the brain affecting emotions, movements and the sensations of pleasure and pain. With taking sugary foods regularly, a tolerance is established that triggers to eat more sugar to derive similar kind of reward which culminates into addiction over time as we continuously feel good. That is the reason why sugar is equated to the effect that drugs like cocaine have on the brain.

It is recommended by the World Health Organisation that men ought to consume nine (9) teaspoons, women six (6) teaspoons while children should have four (4) teaspoons of sugar per day, but this amount has far been surpassed to an extent where people take 30 teaspoons or more per day.

Sugar is seen as a deadly poison, like John Yudkin says in his book, *Pure, White and Deadly*, highlighting that there is no physiological requirement for sugar and that people need not to take sugar to enjoy a completely healthy and nutritious diet. Sugar simply has no nutritional value and does not contain any important micronutrients like minerals and vitamins. It harms the body with immense metabolic disorders and ailments like chronic inflammation, some cancers, diabetes, obesity and cardiovascular diseases. Sugar is hidden in various foods we purchase from the grocery store and so, it is critical to pay attention to food labels and nutritional information of the many discretionary foods we eat every day. It is usually found in foods under different names, but it is still sugar; names such as maltose, dextrose, sucrose, glucose, fructose, lactose and many others. It is very difficult for most people to do away with sugar (that is added sugar). So, the best we can do is to minimise it and indeed get it from intrinsic sources like fruits and vegetables, nuts, legumes and others.

Little nutritional value

It is also evident that highly processed foods have little nutritional value and therefore little levels of vitamins and minerals. Deficiency in these micronutrients deprives someone of the vital function fighting things like free radicals which could easily be deterred by the presence of phytonutrients and antioxidants found in plants. Antioxidants like beta-carotene, lycopene, alpha-carotene, lutein, manganese, vitamins C, vitamin E, vitamin A and selenium, are important to prevent damage of the cells and these can be found in most coloured plants.

Loaded with Trans fats

Ever heard of trans fats? These are fats that are unsaturated, but act like fats that are saturated. Their molecules are fundamentally dissimilar from other kinds of fats, such as Omega-6 and Omega-3 Fatty Acids. The method that certain oils and fats undergo during production, brings about synthetic or mechanically manufactured trans fats. These fats are believed to increase levels of our cholesterol and this ultimately raises our risk of cardiovascular disease. Most highly processed foods are processed using trans fats and eating too much of this has an antagonistic effect on our health. The body fails to break down these kinds of fats, and therefore, they find themselves in an individual's liver and arteries where they become catastrophic. Scientific evidence shows that trans fats *stimulate inflammation* in the body and harm the *endothelial cells* in our blood vessels such as arteries.

Foods high in trans fats include vegetable shortening (*shortening is any type of fat that is solid at room temperature*), microwave popcorn, some margarines, vegetable oils, bakery products, non-diary coffee creamers and so on. It can also be found in foods that are deeply fried and foods that are baked such as cakes, buns biscuits and pastries. Tiny quantities of trans fats are naturally there in veal, lamb, dairy products, mutton and beef.

Too much Salt

Most of the processed food also contain a lot of salt. Yes, salt is indispensable for our existence, but taking too much of it may be detrimental to health. Salt comprises sodium and chloride. The part of the *sodium* is what is considered harmful if taken in excess. Eating too much sodium, mostly from highly refined foods, like biscuits, muffins, cakes, pizza, burgers, pasta, processed meat such as sausages, bacon, polony, some poultry, bread, cereals and some grains, can bring about complications like high blood pressure and heart disease.

Lack of Fibre

Dietary fibre is classified under carbohydrates (starch) which is not digested in the body. Vegetables and fruits have most of the fibre, just as well as in legumes, grains, seeds and nuts. This starch can be *soluble, insoluble* or *resistant*. All these are critical in enhancing good health and lack of one or altering the composition of one may bring about malfunction. Therefore, fibre must work in symbiosis, as a package. This fibre assists in controlling our cholesterol, it helps in controlling our blood sugar, it controls our satiety, it is used as a prebiotic, (that is the food to feed good bacteria, the probiotic), it plays a fundamental part in preventing colorectal cancer and is cardinal in bowel movements. As it reaches the colon undigested, it provides bacteria in the gut ample time to devour it, which is beneficial as the compounds produced largely benefit the body. The good bacteria ferment the fibre forming Short-Chain Fatty Acids (SCFAs, methane, hydrogen and carbon dioxide, as by-products. The SCFAs are subsequently used by the body and feed the good bacteria that ultimately protect us from cancer. Fibre promotes the slow absorption of glucose and fructose found in food and this delay helps thwart blood sugar levels from spiking.

Processed food is deprived of this fibre or has little of it, because fibre does not promote the extended shelf life of the food. Fresh real food is supposed to be eaten at a particular time and not remain on a shelf for long. The body badly needs this fibre and most of the diseases can be prevented if only we ate our appropriate amounts of fibre in our food.

Omega ratios

There must be a decent balance of both Omega-6 (*Linoleic*) and Omega-3 (*Alpha Linolenic*) Fatty Acids. Omega-3 fats are essential fats that must be derived from the diet. They are important for the heart, brain and metabolism. Foods that have these fats are flaxseeds (linseed), chia seeds, sardines, salmon, walnuts, mackerel, anchovies…Omega-6 Fatty Acids are necessary for acute *inflammation* and energy for the body, though these are now eaten in excess causing a lot of trouble. Some examples are sunflower, corn oil, soybean oil, mayonnaise, cashew nuts and almonds. There are also what are known as Omega-9 fats. These are considered non-essential, due to the fact that the body is able to make them. But some diets do still have them such as avocado oil, peanut oil, olive oil, almond oil and cashew nut oil.

Unfortunately, processed food contains very little Omega-3 Fatty Acids. The body transforms these Acids into anti-inflammatory compounds. But too much of the Omega-6 Fatty Acids become *pro-inflammatory*. The ratio of Omega-3 to that of Omega-6 Fatty Acids in our food should preferably be one to one. However, characteristically most of our modern diets are estimated to have Omega-6 to Omega-3 ratio of 25 to 1. This state of affairs promotes a proinflammatory condition in the body that leads to oxidative stress as well as body cell damage.

Dryness

Most highly processed foods are equally very dry. This is the reason why most of the health personnel will recommend that you drink a lot of water in a day, which water does little taken in that manner. The basic reason is that due to the fact that most processed foods are dry, you have to drink a lot of water to make them wet, chewable and assimilable. The foods, as already observed, also contain too much sugar and salt. These compounds require water upon taking them, especially salt that has an effect on the increased levels of water in the body, forming a disequilibrium. If you think about it, you will realise that once you eat more fruits and vegetables, you rarely or not at all crave to drink water, because fruits and vegetables have enough water that is together with other important micronutrients.

Acidity

Most of the highly refined foods are highly acidic, such as products from animals and fast foods. The body is created to optimally work within a certain range and you want to be on the alkaline side, with a blood pH of around 7.3, 7.4. Eating more acidic foods, pushes you out of balance and promotes bad bacteria, viruses and things like cancer cells. It is estimated that it takes more than 20 times the alkalinity amount to counterbalance to acidic environment. The challenge is that we are taking more acidic foods than alkaline ones that contribute heavily to body imbalances.

Inflammatory

Inflammation is a normal procedure that assists the body to defend and heal itself from damage, infection, illness or injury. In response, the body enhances the production of immune cells, cytokines and white blood cells, to assist in the fight against infection. Short-term or acute inflammation could manifest as redness, pain, heat and swelling. Nevertheless, inflammation that is long-term or chronic takes place in our bodies asymptomatically, which can trigger ailments like heart disease, liver cirrhosis, cancer and diabetes. Apart from lifestyle factors, highly refined or processed foods, like refined sugar, are predominantly damaging and can lead to insulin resistance, obesity and diabetes. Scientists say even refined carbohydrates like white flour (white bread), may contribute to systemic inflammation. Vegetable oils, excessive intake of alcohol and processed meats, like polony, are all associated with increased and chronic inflammation.

Excess additives

Almost all highly refined and highly processed foods have additives. Certain chemicals may be added to food to keep it fresh, for colour enhancement, add flavour or texture and indeed make them last longer on the shelf. Such chemicals may include flavour enhancers (such as MSG), food colourings (such as tartrazine or cochineal), or a range of preservatives, flavourants and colourants. The most probable place to find the listing of these additives is on the food or product label. They are normally listed in a descending order by weight with a few exceptions on flavourants. They can be represented by a code or labelled in full.

Individuals differ in the manner they react to food additives, such as having a rash, diarrhoea or other food reactions. Despite the fact that food industries use many additives in food, that are equally there in nature, too much of the industrial additives have raised debate and concerns on the health of consumers. Additives can come in many different forms and use. It could be through artificial sweeteners, colours, flavours and flavour enhancers, foaming agents, mineral salts, raising agents, flour treatment to improve baking quality, preservatives, thickeners and vegetable gums. Food additives may indeed cause hypersensitivity such as nervous disorders, skin problems, digestive disorders and respiratory ailments.

Healthy Claims

Highly processed food in the middle aisles (mostly) of the supermarket has so much health claims. The health claims are statements made by the food industries during advertising and on the food labels. These could be talking about having more fibre, lowering cholesterol, low or no sugar, low or no fat, good source of potassium and so on. The food in this section is usually packaged and has so much writings on the package. The *talking* seems non-stop and very convincing. Some of the foods *talking to you* have more than five additives and ingredients and others can go up to 15, with unpronounceable names. The main reason for most of these kinds of foods is convenience, because they are foods that are mostly ready-to-eat, are cheaper and not much re-cooking is required. You can eat them there and then. Contrast this with real whole food in the fresh food section which does not claim anything.

PROMINENT CHRONIC DISEASES OF CONCERN

In as far as the World Health Organisation is concerned, Chronic illnesses or Non-Communicable Diseases (NCDs), (others call them degenerative diseases), kill about 41 million people annually, which translates to 71% of all deaths globally. Coronary artery disease, diabetes, cancer and stroke feature prominently as critical diseases presenting havoc and causing premature deaths. People of the ages 30 and 69, account for about 15 million deaths annually, with most of them from low-and-middle-income countries. As the name implies, NCDs cannot be transmissible directly from one person to another and they also take long to resurface. Their prevalence is associated with many factors such as lifestyle, food and nutrition, genetics, physical and psychological factors.

The occurrence of chronic illness brings about lack of basic necessities as it entails poverty in developing countries, particularly by upping coasts at household level in line with healthcare. Susceptible and socially deprived persons tend to be ill and may pass away faster than persons that are higher on the social strata in society. Healthcare costs for chronic illnesses rapidly drain household resources. The excessive costs of chronic disease, including often prolonged and expensive treatment and loss of an individual who is the main source of income, force millions of people into poverty annually and hinder personal and national development. Most Governments' health expenditures have more than doubled in recent years, to address the challenges brought about by the presence of Non-Communicable Diseases.

In the current scenario, you could either be affected by the prevalence of chronic diseases or indeed you could be one of the people suffering from such illnesses. This is so because research keeps narrowing the gap-ratio of people suffering from chronic diseases and every day, the ratio is getting closer to you and me. In most developed countries, it is estimated that one in three people suffer from such ailments. So, in a set up where you are with two of your friends right now, it is estimated that one of you has it. That's pretty close!

Forget about the traditional thought that these diseases only affect the old and the rich people. Children and their parents, grandparents, the rich and the poor are all susceptible to the risk factors contributing to chronic diseases. Based on some of those highlighted factors, everyone is at risk. Scientists and researchers have done and keep doing massive epidemiological and experimental research on the matters surrounding chronic illness and one common and sure denominator is that diet and lifestyle play a critical and huge role in the prevalence of non-communicable diseases.

Unhealthy diets and a sedentary life may manifest in what is known as metabolic risk factors (or metabolic syndrome, also called syndrome x), that come through elevated blood glucose (hyperglycaemia), high blood pressure, or excess levels of fat (hyperlipidaemia), abnormal cholesterol and triglyceride levels and obesity. Syndrome x actually is a constellation of disorders that take place at the same time, triggering the occurrence of Type 2 diabetes, stroke and heart disease, which are among the leading chronic diseases that cause massive deaths.

In this book, am more concerned with the unhealthy diets, as highlighted in the preceding chapter on highly processed or refined foods and sedentary or lack of physical activity associated with chronic diseases. Among the kernel of this chapter are stroke, heart disease, high blood pressure, diabetes, obesity and cancer. According to research and WHO, the leading metabolic risk factor for most people globally is raised blood pressure which is said to account for about 20% of deaths globally. Then comes obesity and hyperglycaemia or elevated glucose in the blood.

High Blood Pressure (HBP)

Blood is an important component of the body. It is found everywhere in our bodies. The heart pumps the blood in and throughout our bodies. As this goes on, the pressure thrusting beside the blood vessel walls fluctuates. As the heart pushes blood in arteries, there is usually excessive pressure and when it is relaxed, there is minimal pressure. The Blood Pressure (BP), therefore, denotes the two readings; the highest (*systolic*) over the lowest (*diastolic*). The systolic reading occurs when the blood pressure in arteries makes the heart *contract* and it's the higher number on top of the reading, while diastolic is when the pressure of the blood in arteries makes the heart *relax*, filled with blood. This is the bottom number on the reading of BP.

That which may be considered a healthy blood pressure differs from person to person. This disease rarely gives warning signals because one could have raised blood pressure and feel perfectly fine, unless it is checked. That is why HBP is seen among the *deadliest silent killers*. As far as Low Blood Pressure (LBP) is concerned, it is relative because what could be considered low for one individual may be quite alright for another individual. Challenges only arise when it has a harmful effect on the body affecting your health.

The blood pressure naturally rises and falls all the time, in line with what the heart needs and also dependent on your activities. If someone is told that he or she has HBP, it implies that his or her pressure is insistently higher than is normal. There is also what is known as *white coat hypertension*, or *white coat syndrome*, which is a spectacle in which someone displays a blood pressure level above the normal range, because they are in the doctor's office for example, which is different when they are not. It is thought that such occurrences may be due to nervousness of being at the hospital.

Chronic raised BP is among the cardinal danger factors associated with various ailments such as stroke, kidney malfunction and heart diseases. The normal or optimal blood pressure is usually 120/80mmHg and may go up to 129/84mmHg to be still considered normal. The pressure of the blood is said to be elevated if one registers a reading greater than 140/90 mmHg, posing a threat for a heart attack or stroke. In medical terms, this is called *Hypertension*, worsened if it becomes chronic.

The following is only a guide on various readings of blood pressure:

- *Normal blood pressure*: at or lower than 120/80 mmHg.
- *Raised Blood Pressure*: systolic reading at 120 to 129 mmHg; while that of diastolic lower at 80 mmHg. Raised pressure may worsen, unless addressed.
- *Stage 1 hypertension*. Systolic as at 130 to 139 mmHg; diastolic pressure, 80 to 89 mmHg.
- *Stage 2 hypertension*: severe raised pressure; Systolic at 140 mmHg even above or that of diastolic at 90 mmHg or higher.

Elevated pressure of the blood is not known how exactly it comes about, but it may be strongly influenced by factors like obesity, level of physical activity, genetics, lifestyle, diet, stress, anxiety, smoking and excess alcohol consumption. It is argued that some medicines can also elevate blood pressure. Eating too much sodium from salt is also considered among the triggers of HBP, because most of this sodium consumed, isn't put as you eat food, but it is concealed in highly refined food, eaten daily such as in canned food, cereals, cakes, pasta and pizza.

Elevated pressure of the blood is associated with cardiovascular diseases by injuring and deteriorating walls of the blood vessels. It can equally bring about blood clots or atheroma breaking off walls of the arteries and block an artery in the brain as well as ingest heart disease complications. It can silently destroy the body for many years before symptoms come up. If it is not diagnosed and controlled, the affected person may incur a disability, poor health or even a deadly stroke or heart attack.

Arteries that are healthy are accommodating, resilient and flexible and their interior inside layer is smooth to allow for free flow of blood, providing essential tissues and organs with oxygen and nutrients. But HBP steadily rises the pressure in the arteries resulting in arteries that are narrowed and damaged. Once bad fats from your food, such as trans fats, get into the bloodstream, they may accumulate in the ravaged arteries. Ultimately, the walls of the artery reduce in elasticity, restricting the easy flow of blood. On the other hand, the brain relies on a healthful supply of blood to function appropriately and endure, but HBP may bring forth mini strokes or a transitory interruption of supply of blood to the brain, scientifically known as transient ischemic stroke. Elevated pressure may equally damage the blood vessels in the kidneys leading to *nephropathy* among others. Add diabetes to high blood pressure, the destruction might be insurmountable.

Eyes might also be affected by HBP. The small, sensitive vessels that supply blood to the eye could be harmed. Further, it is estimated that problems with erection get progressively widespread more especially when men are in their 50s. This could be worsened with the presence of elevated pressure of blood. Consequently, soaring blood pressure is associated with damaging blood vessel linings, causing stiffened and narrowed arteries which will limit the flow of blood. For women, high blood pressure can decrease the flow of blood to the vagina and may diminish sexual arousal and/or desire, vagina becoming dry or trouble reaching orgasm. It may also cause bone loss by increasing the amount of calcium in the urine leading to osteoporosis (loss of bone mass), that may eventually bring about bone fractures. Older women are more at risk. One may also experience sleep disorder such as Obstructive Sleep Apnoea (OSA), where your throat muscles relax causing loud snoring.

Alternatively, a way of life that is healthier, which would include good nutrition and staying active, are among key remedies to raised blood pressure. Doing regular physical activity, trying to stop smoking, reducing salt in your diet, eating adequate amounts of fruit and vegetables, avoiding being obese and appropriate intake of alcohol in a day [that is two (2) drinks for men and one (1) drink, women], are among key things to do. You should also have enough sleep, avoid stress, depression and brain fog. For some people in acute situations, they may still require drugs to assist lower the levels of blood pressure to suitable ones. Although drugs are generally helpful at decreasing blood pressure, they heal symptoms and may instigate side-effects in some individuals.

A plant-based nutrient dense approach is important to consider here, just as it works on many other illnesses. Dietary Approach to Stopping Hypertension (DASH), stresses the need to eat more vegetables, fruits, oily fish, legumes, nuts and whole grains among others. People with HBP are advised to minimise their intake of things like sugar and salt. In terms of salt, this operates on the kidneys to retain more water. The retained water increases the blood pressure and places stress on the heart, arteries, brain and the kidneys themselves. Therefore, reducing the amount of salt in the food is considered a better way to tackle raised blood pressure. It may also help blood pressure medicines like diuretics, to work well. Nevertheless, it is not easy to do this most times because most of the salt is concealed in the highly processed foods that we eat all the times.

Heart Diseases

Scientists and researchers estimate that every 29 minutes, someone somewhere dies of heart disease. Heart disease is a generic name for a range of conditions that concern the heart. Some people may say *cardiovascular disease* while others use the term *heart disease.* They are talking about the same thing, except that in cardiovascular disease, it generally denotes circumstances that consist of reduced or obstructed blood vessels that may culminate not only into a heart attack, but also stroke. The other forms of heart conditions, like those that involve the valves or rhythm and the heart muscle, are also part of what heart disease is.

The heart works every day, every minute and throughout the year. It does not go on break or vacation like some other organs would, because if it did, then you would be near-dead or dead indeed. It is estimated that our hearts will beat about 3 billion times, should we live an average lifetime. So, having a healthy heart, through prevention and management, would probably be one of the most important health decisions you will ever make in your life.

Among the many situations that include the heart is what is referred to as coronary heart disease, heart failure, heart attack, angina (chest pains), arrhythmias (abnormal heart beats), peripheral vascular disease (an illness of the big vessels of blood like the feet, legs and arms), congenital heart illness (imperfections or deformities of the heart or blood vessels prior to birth), septal defect (irregular opening amid right and left sides of the heart), rheumatic heart ailment (fever and mostly distressing the valves of the heart) and aneurysm, (a swelling instigated by waning of the artery or muscle of the heart).

Blood is pumped by the heart, in particular getting it from the entire body and pumping it to the lungs for oxygenation. Thence, from the lungs, it is presented as red blood, because in it, there is oxygen. From there, the blood that is oxygenated, is accordingly pumped to the entire body. Heart disease or heart attacks have something to do with clog-up of arteries that carry oxygenated blood to the heart. When we talk about heart disease and clogged arteries, it is not the arteries that take blood from the heart to the entire body. These are *coronary arteries*, primarily providing the heart with blood, because the heart is actually a muscle in itself and therefore requires oxygenated blood as well.

So, over time, you may develop *atheroma* or *plaques* that build-up alongside artery walls, if for example, you do not have an appropriate diet, alcoholism, smoking or you have a susceptibility to it. The atheroma and the substance therein could be cholesterol, dead white cells or fat, that form a messy substance. The development of the plaque hinders the blood vessels, that essentially blocks the arteries. This is referred to as *Atherosclerosis*. Once these plagues build up, they may eventually narrow the actual vessel that is supplying blood to the heart. Blood would be obstructed and in that general process, there will be limitation of the flow of blood, that is now what is called *Ischemia*, which is simply the lack of oxygen and blood flow to the heart. This brings about *coronary artery disease*, or *heart disease*. They are referred to as *coronary arteries* due to the fact that they *surround* the heart muscle in the way of a *crown*. The term *coronary* is Latin derived, *corona* and there is also Greek, *koron* implying *crown*. Therefore, to say *coronary heart disease* becomes unnecessary, as *coronary* is in fact already talking about the heart.

Back. If the heart is not receiving all the oxygen it needs, particularly while exerting oneself or exercising, you require extra oxygen and the heart demands pumping slightly more, possibly raising blood pressure. In this condition, the cells in the heart are not receiving the oxygen needed, so, the heart might not be in a position to deliver all of the tasks accordingly. When that happens, that is what brings about the condition called *heart failure,* being among the triggers of heart disease. In this condition (heart failure), it does not necessarily mean that the heart has stopped working and the person is dead, but it simply means that the heart is not managing to perform according to expectation. It is indeed not able to *take care of* the requirements of that individual and therefore, not pumping adequately or accordingly to deliver sufficient work.

Like stated earlier, additional symptoms that indeed may take place when an individual has coronary artery disease, where they have a blockage, is *Ischemia,* which is the deprivation of oxygen to the heart muscle. In this state, the person may feel some strangulation and pain called *Angina Pectoris* or simply *angina.* This is literally chest pain. Angina refers to the strangulation and Pectoris refers to the chest.

This is not a desirable condition because the body is not working as expected. Some plaques are actually unstable and they keep growing making heart disease worse. When the plaque is not stable, it may grow big and may actually rupture, necessitated by the turbulent blood flow. When it ruptures, the contents of the plaque, (that is the lipid, the dead white blood cells or the cholesterol) are subjected to the flow of blood, specifically to the clotting-factor. This is extremely *thrombogenic* matter, as it has a tendency to bring about blood-clots. Thrombosis is all about blood clotting. When this occurs, it begins to overly inhibit the blood vessels and every so often, it may entirely hamper the vessel. With this condition, you are substantially diminishing the flow of blood to the heart and might even be shutting it off. Consequently, the cells in the heart will no longer get oxygen and they may die, in what is termed as *infarction*. An *infarct* is in reality a heart tissue that is dead.

When the tissue of the heart starts to die, as in *infarct,* this is adverse than what was described earlier in heart failure. Not only where the heart is getting inadequate oxygen, but in this case, the cells are truly dead. This challenge of entirely or virtually denying cells of oxygen and they die, is scientifically called *myocardial infarction* or in lay man's terms, a *heart attack.* Myocardial implies the dying of the tissue of the heart muscle. It is less likely. However, sometimes a plaque could also be present and develop a thromboembolism. It could be this thrombogenic material and clots with it that would essentially go and block the artery in this embolism manner. That may also block arteries and affect the tissue that would die. But the key trigger is this extreme clotting that can happen quite rapidly and totally have the artery blocked.

So, take note that *heart attack* is not *cardiac arrest.* An individual may be affected by a heart attack and could have portions of their muscle tissue dead or infarct. This is not referred to as cardiac arrest, because you may have some part of your heart tissue collapsed or dead, but you could still stay alive. Your heart would be compromised, but you could live on. *Cardiac arrest* is precisely your entire heart ceasing to work because it dies, which would lead to eventual death. A dreadful heart attack and starving heart tissue of oxygen, may trigger infarction leading to cardiac arrest. Take note however, that a heart attack will not all the time lead to cardiac arrest and that a heart attack may not be the only way that can bring about cardiac arrest.

When the blood vessels have narrowed due to build-up of plague, in medical terms, that is called *stenosis.* For example, if a person goes to exercise and his cardiac muscle cells need oxygen, he would probably not be able to get the needed oxygen because of the stenosis which caused ischemia. Because of that, the cells will not be able to help the heart pump properly and this therefore may lead to heart failure, where the heart is failing to correctly do its function and not entirely shutting down. Because of this disease, the muscle cells in the heart really need to pump hard during strenuous exercise and the heart will not be able to do it because it is not getting enough oxygen.

Some risk factors associated with heart disease include being obese or overweight, smoking, not exercising, a bad diet, excess alcohol and stress. The circumstances that impinge on blood circulation, like elevated cholesterol, blood pressure, diabetes and atrial fibrillation (heartbeat that's not regular), also exacerbate the danger of Coronary Artery Disease (CAD).

Stroke

Brain cells need a steady and continuous provision of nutrients and oxygenated blood, like the case is for the heart and other organs. This is accomplished through a structure of vessels of blood that get to all parts of the brain. When all of a sudden there is an interruption, the cells in the brain start to die. This damage is called a stroke.

The way a stroke happens is very similar to the condition of coronary artery disease. Stroke is also considered part of the cardiovascular diseases. Strokes are grave health ailments that happen when the supply of the blood to some brain parts are disrupted. Similar to the heart, the brain requires important nutrients and oxygen in the blood to suitably work. If blood supply is constrained or indeed halted, the cells of the brain may die leading to brain damage and possible death. That is an emergency and swift measures are vital at this time.

So, strokes involve the brain; with a rapid loss of its function due to something odd taking place with the flow of the blood. Two (2) major types of strokes are worth talking about: *Ischemic* and *Haemorrhagic*. These can be further sub-categorised.

In ischemia, most strokes do take place when a clot of the blood gets stuck in some brain arteries, obstructing the flow of the blood. In some instances, the clot is made within the artery which is called a *thrombotic stroke*. Or indeed, a blood clot or a dense form of wreckage, starting from somewhere else gets to the brain and breaks the artery of the brain in what is known as an *embolic stroke*.

Various portions of the brain perform various functions and thence the signs and symptoms of stroke may differ. This could be eminent in movement, speech, sight, sensation, coordination or balance. At times, a stroke may take place before what is known as a *Transient Ischemic Attacks* (TIAs), which are short-term occurrences or mini strokes and may take a few minutes to several hours. Such kind usually vanish on their own, but havoc maybe building up inside.

From the description of heart diseases and the condition of stenosis and ischemia and heart attacks, *Ischemia* is a shortage of the flow of blood to specific tissues of the body. Therefore, ischemic stroke is comparable to the condition in a heart attack, except that here, it is not taking place in a coronary blood vessel, but in a blood vessel in the brain. If there is a large clot of the blood that forms in some brain part, it might be due to plaques that possibly ruptured. Whichever way, the blood clot restricts the blood flow and this clot is a thrombus, or that thrombosis has occurred. The brain tissue that is further after the clot will not receive its oxygen and may die or indeed suffer infarction. This is the reason why ischemic strokes are at times known as *cerebral infarctions*. Most strokes occur as ischemic ones, an estimated 87% of all strokes.

The other means in which someone may be affected by ischemia in the vessels of the blood, is by thromboembolism. This a clot of the blood that gets broken off and develops into an embolus. Due to the fact that it is an embolus because of a blood clot, that is why it is called thromboembolism, which eventually blocks an artery. So, when we talk about *thrombus*, it implies a clot of blood formed in the vein, whilst an *embolus* is whatever treks all the way through the vessels of blood until it gets to a vessel that is too tiny to let it go. Once this takes place, the *embolus* halts the flow of blood. Blood flow gets blocked yonder the brain, that may instigate infarction, rendering the brain tissue dead. That distinct tissue of the brain and its mental function could make it incredibly difficult for the individual undergoing a stroke to perform some tasks.

It is not every time visible that someone has a stroke, which may be referred to as a *silent stroke*, but destruction is still happening. According to medical information, the individual suffering a stroke might not even realise that harm is happening. He or she may simply have severe pain, or he or she may be unable to appropriately move about a side of the body, or that of the face, or unable to correctly speak. It actually varies according to what component of the brain is being injured. However, in either of these conditions, ischemic stroke is initiated by some form of blood restriction or obstruction that affects the brain receiving inadequate oxygen, which might cause cells to die.

The other type of stroke is *Haemorrhagic*. To *haemorrhage* means *to bleed*. Therefore, for haemorrhagic stroke, blood vessel would fundamentally crack. It is deeply correlated with *high blood pressure* and other risk considerations. If a blood vessel snaps, in this manner, all the blood would be spilling into the brain in a hysterical manner. The blood pouring into the brain hysterically like this, will muddle some part of the brain, (say a part with neurons that transmit information to other nerve cells) and this may cause some parts to die. It would also affect the flow of blood to be diminished, depriving cells further up inability to receive oxygenated blood required, as all the blood is being splashed all over. Because 87% of strokes are thought to be ischemic, the remaining 13% is therefore haemorrhagic.

It is advisable to look for certain signs and symptoms for stroke-affected persons in what researchers and studies call *B.E.F.A.S.T*:

- *Balance* – how well the persons is balancing.
- *Eyes* – the state of the eyes must be checked.
- *Face* – Examine their face, if their mouth sagged.
- *Arms* – Trying to lift both arms.
- *Speech* – Check for incoherent speech and how they understand you.
- *Time* – Is critical, which is the period of stroke and action.

If any of the above signs and symptoms are evident or you are suspicious that you or another person may be having a stroke, call or action for emergency.

Just like the case with heart disease, risk factors for stroke include obese or overweight, smoking, not exercising, a bad diet, excess alcohol and stress. The circumstances that impinge on blood circulation, like elevated cholesterol, blood pressure, diabetes and atrial fibrillation (heartbeat that's not regular), also exacerbate the dangers of a stroke.

Cancer

Cancer refers to a group of interconnected illnesses. In all forms of cancer, some of the cells of the body start to divide with no control and disperse into nearby tissues. The cells of cancer are less specialised than normal cells because as typical cells get fully grown into very distinctive types of cells with particular purposes, cancer cells don't. They go on to divide ceaselessly. Additionally, the cancer cells manage to overlook signals that usually tell cells to stop splitting or that start a procedure called *apoptosis,* which is programmed cell death. The body uses apoptosis to get rid of unwanted cells. Cancer wrecks damage to genes brought about by cancer causing elements. The elements that cause cancer are called *carcinogens* which could be a chemical substance, from smoking or indeed an environmental, viral or genetic factor.

Cancer, therefore, is a state in which body *cells* in a specific section of the body develop and *replicate without control.* The carcinogenic cells can damage adjacent healthy tissues, together with organs. Often times, cancer begins in one area of the body before spreading to other parts. This process is known as *metastasis.* Cancer's early signs and symptoms are variations to the body's typical processes or signs and symptoms that are extraordinary. For instance, an abrupt appearance of a lump on the body, baffling bleeding or changes to your digestive system, could all be attributed to cancer and may need attention.

Trillions of cells make up our bodies and cancer can begin almost from anyplace in the body such as the reproductive organs, lungs, intestines, skin, blood and the breast. Ordinarily, the cells of the body develop and split to produce brand new cells as the body requires them. When cells grow old or get damaged, they die and new cells take up their place. When cancer cells develop, nonetheless, this systematic process collapses. As cells turn out to be more and more abnormal, old or damaged cells stay alive when they are supposed to die and new cells develop when they are not required. These additional cells can divide devoid of stopping and may produce growths called *tumours.* Tumours are abnormal growth of cells that serve no function. Many cancers produce strong tumours, which are throngs of tissue.

When you go to the hospital with suspected cancer, the physicians will first of all try to find out whether you have *benign* or *malignant tumours.* In literal sense, malignant is cancerous and benign is non-cancerous.

In this regard, cancerous tumours are said to be *malignant* if they do proliferate into, or damage, adjacent tissues. Additionally, as the tumours expand, some cancer cells can detach themselves and move to faraway parts in the body via the lymph system or blood and develop new tumours far from the initial tumour. In breasts, for instance, cancer starts within the breast tissue itself and may spread to lymph nodes in the armpit with delayed diagnosis and treatment. Once breast cancer is in the lymph nodes, the tumours move to some other body parts, like bones, liver and so on. These cancer cells can then form tumours in those places.

As opposed to malignant tumours, *benign tumours* don't multiply into, or attack, adjacent tissues, but instead they can sometimes be pretty big. When benign tumours are removed, they normally do not develop back, which is different from malignant tumours that do at times. So, malignant tumours are not benign tumours because the latter are not cancerous, as they do not attack close- by tissues or spread to other body parts the way cancerous ones do. But they can also be a serious concern if they exert on important areas like blood vessels and nerves. They can come about due to unknown reasons but could also be through genetics, diet, trauma, stress, toxins and inflammation or infection as well as some use of certain drugs.

Some of the most common cancers are:

❖ Lung
❖ Prostate
❖ Cervical
❖ Breast
❖ Skin
❖ Colon
❖ Rectal

- ❖ Ovarian
- ❖ Carcinoma
- ❖ Head and Neck
- ❖ Uterine
- ❖ Sarcoma
- ❖ Lymphoma
- ❖ Leukaemia
- ❖ Thyroid
- ❖ Melanoma

It is argued that just a minor percentage of all cancers in humans are related to solely genetic influences. The rest of the cancers consist of peripheral or exterior influences, such as food and nutrition. Studies show that no one factor would be singled out as the cause of cancer. Some medications and procedures, are also known to increase cancer risk. Regular screening is recommended to detect cancer, but overall, preventing cancer as priority is even much better through the food we eat and the lifestyle we lead.

Diabetes

Diabetes is a critical and intricate disease which can disturb the whole body. It needs everyday care and if not addressed, can have serious ramifications on the health of an individual causing death. Despite its challenge, one has to make a choice to be happy and work towards reversing the condition. Diabetes comes in different stern and multifaceted textures with the three key ones being Type 1, Type 2 and Gestational Diabetes. If an individual has diabetes, his or her body would not sustain healthy levels of blood sugar or glucose, which is a kind of sugar and the main foundation of energy for the body. Excessive levels of glucose in the blood (especially from carbohydrates like sugar) may have serious health repercussions in the long and short term. For the body to function well, it needs to change glucose from the food we eat to energy and this is successfully accomplished by the hormone *Insulin*. For someone with diabetes, there is no insulin production or indeed the insulin is ineffective.

We have an estimated ten to one-hundred trillion cells. All cells in our bodies need enough energy to endure and perform various roles; it be brain cells that need energy to maintain energising other cells in the brain and transmitting messages and signals; muscle cells that need the strength to contract and do other essential tasks. The main factor from which the cells get the energy is a simple sugar called *glucose*. Glucose actually tastes sweet. It is transported to the cells via the blood stream. In an idyllic situation when the cells require energy, glucose would get into the cells. Regrettably, it is not that straightforward for the big bulk of cells in the human body, as the glucose may not get into the cell by itself. It requires the aid of *insulin*.

On the exterior of cells, there are what are known as *insulin receptors*. For glucose to be assimilated by the cells, insulin ought to attach itself to the receptors, which open the outlets. Insulin must attach to insulin receptors and subsequently, the glucose can be assimilated. So, insulin is like a *key*, working together with its receptors to open the door to the cells. Regrettably, things do not work always as planned or designed, because most times, we choose a different pessimistic path.

Type 1 diabetes is known as an auto-immune disorder where the immune system is triggered to destruct pancreatic cells that produce insulin. How exactly that happens, no one knows. The *beta cells* of the pancreas produce insulin. But then, if the pancreas is not supplying insulin, nothing will bind to the insulin receptors and subsequently, the glucose outlets won't be opened. The glucose will not be able to enter the cells. Therein, you have Type 1 diabetes.

This diabetes starts unknowingly and can include urination, extreme thirst, sudden weight loss, weakness, exhaustion and distorted vision. Individuals suffering from Type 1 diabetes need to insert insulin several times a day or use an insulin pump to stabilise the sugar in their body. With this condition, you have to rely on insulin always for your carbohydrates and check your glucose levels many times during the day. Type 1 diabetes happens most commonly in juveniles, but current trends and research show that more and more people over the age of 30 develop it too.

On the other hand, Type 2 diabetes is a chronic situation where the body gradually becomes insulin resistant and may lose the ability to produce sufficient insulin in the pancreas. Its onset is connected to lifestyle and food risk factors as well as genetic influences. Most people suffering from diabetes nowadays have Type 2 diabetes and can be found in both young and old.

If insulin is being produced by the pancreas and placing it into the bloodstream, it gets used, but a condition could occur where the receptors are not functioning well and they might have been desensitised to insulin. In this situation, the receptors have difficulty binding to the insulin and glucose does not enter the cell. Excess glucose in the blood results and you have what is called *hyperglycaemia*. This scenario is what is typical of Type 2 diabetes.

So, if you have Type 2 diabetes, implies that the pancreas is no longer making adequate insulin, or the insulin being produced is ineffective in that the body is now resistant. *You are insulin resistant.* The opposite of this is *insulin sensitive.* Type 2 diabetes is a disorder that happens over a period of many years and as the body gets to being insulin resistant, the pancreas works harder and harder in order to generate additional insulin to process the glucose in the bloodstream. With time, pancreatic cells can become damaged, whilst the body's opposition to insulin persists and grows.

For Type 2 diabetes, drugs and lifestyle changes may be implored to help resensitise the body to glucose and insulin. Just like with Type 1, insulin can also be injected into the bloodstream in Type 2, because even if the cells are desensitised, it does not mean they will not bind with insulin; it just means it will take more insulin to uptake the same amount of glucose. Adding enough insulin, therefore, may be adequate to attach to insulin receptors and bring about absorption of glucose.

Remember, cells won't function without glucose, but excess sugar in the bloodstream may essentially trigger a lot of destruction to the body.

Obesity

Obesity could be considered as a condition linked with disproportionate body fat that aggravates the danger of health complications. It is not a disease per say. It is an abnormal and excessive fat accumulation, a condition or disorder that may trigger a chain of chronic illnesses. It is a word used in defining an individual who could be extremely obese with a high notch of fat in the body. Excess weight would be key here and may have adversative impact.

Obesity is known to generate a number of chronic disorders. Fat which is placed in the body may be more than the energy we use in various activities and when we are sedentary. Minor disproportions for some time may bring about more weight or being obese. Together with other persistent illnesses like diabetes, heart disease, stroke and cancer, obesity is estimated to cause over 30 million deaths worldwide. The World Health Organisation (WHO) indicates that obesity and overweight are the main dangerous reasons for several non-communicable disorders. They are a challenge in developed countries and the figures are also hugely on the increase in developing countries, predominantly in urban areas.

The distribution of fat is significant when evaluating obesity or overweight and the related disease condition. The common way to measure someone's weight is through the Body Mass Index (BMI), that is the *weight in kilograms* divided by the *height in metres squared*. Therefore, a BMI:

- between 18 and 25 is deemed normal
- between 25 and 29, is believed to be overweight
- between 30 and 40, seen as obese
- and that over 40, overly or morbidly obese

You can also use other methods to determine risk, such as waist circumference and other methods. Waist perimeter or circumference exceeding 94 cm for men and beyond 80 cm for women is thought to be overweight and an indicator of severe chronic risk of disease. The waist circumference more than 102 cm for men and about 88 cm for women is viewed as obese.

As hinted earlier, obesity intensifies the risk of many chronic and hypothetical deadly sicknesses. Largely, the more body fat one has, the higher the health risk. Take note that the volume of weight added during adulthood period, does add to the complications. Obesity is linked with diseases such as stroke, gout, sleep apnoea, insulin resistance, high blood pressure, heart disease, some cancers, Type 2 diabetes, gall bladder syndrome, cataracts, polycystic ovarian syndrome, among others.

Obesity may be caused by childhood risk considerations and puberty, because a high number of obese youngsters and young people grow up to be obese grownups. According to Dr. Robert Lustig, in his book, *"Fat Chance..." human fat cells are defined at the age of two for almost all individuals.*

Obesity is also associated with a sedentary life, eating highly refined or processed foods, stress, lack of adequate sleep and to some extent, genetic factors.

Dementia and Alzheimer's

Dementia is a cluster of brain disorders that inhibit thinking and everyday functioning. The dementia symptoms are triggered by syndromes involving the brain and it's not a particular illness. Just as you might have heart attack or brain attack, dementia could be considered a *mind attack* because it impacts on the behaviour and affects the capacity to do daily and normal functions. The brain function is affected such that the person's usual social or normal life is interrupted. The disease is prominent among the older population, but it can also be seen in the younger ones. There are several types of dementia with their own causes. The most common forms of dementia are Alzheimer's disease, Fronto Temporal Lobar Degeneration (FTLD), Huntington's disease, Vascular dementia, Alcohol related dementia (Korsakoff's syndrome), Dementia with Lewy bodies and Creutzfeldt-Jacob disease. Although it can be genetic, most types of dementia are not.

Alzheimer's

Alzheimer's is a progressive particular type of dementia and is characterised by brain syndrome that produces problems with thinking, memory and behaviour in mostly the grownups. The condition affects millions of people, mostly in developed countries, although the developing world is quickly catching up. It is mostly used as a substitute for overall or umbrella term *dementia*. It is estimated that between 50-70% of all dementia cases, are actually Alzheimer's.

Dr. Alois Alzheimer, a German neurologist described the first case of Alzheimer's in 1906, identifying two major physical attributes of the ailment when he analysed the tissue of a brain of a woman under a microscope after her death. He discovered abnormal protein clusters and tangled bundles of nerve fibres. Studies indicate that four factors are observed in the brain tissue of a dead individual from Alzheimer's; the two as noted above and also inflammation and loss of nerve cell.

The prominent presence of plaque, which is a protein deposit that develops in the areas between nerve cells, is extensively thought to be what begins the disorder in the brain. Bent *tangles* of proteins called *tau proteins* may develop inside the nerve cells and along with an amplified number of *plaques*, which may block interaction between nerve cells. The continuous failure for the link between nerve cells, destroys them such that they may no longer work accordingly in memory regions of the brain. The cells of the nerve ultimately die. As more nerve cells die, brain components that control language, thinking skills and reasoning equally get affected and brain tissue starts to dwindle. Scientists and researchers also believe that chronic inflammation performs a crucial role in the development of Alzheimer's.

Once this happens, the person will have trouble to remember newly acquired info or knowledge, like recent discussions, people's names or events. However, not all people will exhibit these symptoms from the onset as some people may first develop behavioural variations, language complications or sight problems. Some might experience forgetting appointments, questioning over and over, repeating statements, expressing thoughts or participating in conversations, regularly losing possessions, forgetting names of loved ones, getting lost in familiar places, problems sourcing the right words to identify objects and many more other symptoms.

Alzheimer's is not clear how it comes about. Nevertheless, research shows that the ailment is prompted by a mixture of lifestyle, environment and diet. These may impact negatively on the brain with time. Old age (maybe after 60), is also seen as a major risk factor for Alzheimer's, but this is not exclusive. Other factors could include genetics or family history.

Autoimmune Diseases

An autoimmune disease is triggered by an immune system that attacks its own healthy cells. This disease occurs when the body's immune system is persistently overactive and invades the cells. Ordinarily, our immune system defends our body and works to keep us healthy by resisting infection. However, bacteria and viruses may quickly transform to dodge the immune system. In that regard, our immune system must mutate just as hastily to protect us.

More than 80 different types of autoimmune diseases have been researched and identified and most of them are chronic, with the harshness of the disease fluctuating with time. The diseases are said to mostly affect women more than men and the further away from the equator, the more prominent they become. Some examples of Autoimmune Diseases include Lupus, Coeliac, Rheumatoid Arthritis, Polymyalgia Rheumatica, Sjögren's Syndrome, Multiple Sclerosis, Ankylosing Spondylitis, Grave's Diseases and Type 1 Diabetes.

The element of autoimmunity happens when, instead of attacking viruses, fungi, bacteria and other infections, the immune system attacks healthy organs and tissues. It is not known why this occurs. However, in *Medical Medium*, Anthony Williams argues and emphasises that there is nothing like autoimmunity, because most of such diseases are caused by Epstein-Barr Virus (EBV) and that the body can never attack itself.

Autoimmune conditions may also commonly affect people with a hereditary tendency. Factors such as stress, an infection, diet, radiation, medication and radiation, may be autoimmune symptomatic, just as microbes in the gut might also stimulate the condition. Most people have signs and symptoms of autoimmune condition for some time before they seek medical help. Due to the nature of the diseases, it usually takes a long time to establish and diagnose that one has an autoimmune disease. This is due to the fact that some symptoms, such as tiredness and just *not feeling all right*, are normally experienced by several individuals, which symptoms could vary with time. With most situations, not a single test would easily confirm it.

Although there is no known cure for autoimmunity, individuals may well embark on a good diet that avoids being overweight, avoid sedentary life, sleeping enough and avoiding stressing situations.

WHY PLANT-BASED FOOD?

Prof. Michael Pollan has popularised an important mantra with only seven (7) words, which I love and embrace wholeheartedly: *Eat Food, Not too Much, Mostly Plants*. This means that we need to eat food, *real food*, like vegetables, fruits, whole grains, nuts, seeds, legumes and others. That food should be eaten in moderation (*including moderation*) and that most of it should be plants, as plants contain most of the nutrients we require to stay well and healthy.

Research has showed that more than 95% of the chronic illnesses in our lives, we ourselves are responsible for them and there should be no convincing reason anyone of us should have chronic illnesses such as Stroke, High Blood Pressure, Diabetes, Obesity, Cancer, Heart Disease and Autoimmune Diseases among many. Less than five (5%) percent of the illnesses may be considered genetic illnesses, but there have also been studies and arguments that even genetic ailments can, to a large extent, be addressed or well managed by a plant-based nutrition.

What to eat and not what to eat is a personal choice or decision that we all make all the times. Research and studies estimate that on average, people make more than 15 and up to 200 food and drink decisions per day. But there are certain times when we need to be pushed, reminded or challenged to make proper decisions. And that area is non-other than food and lifestyle. I feel duty bound and responsible to highlight this subject as well, because it borders on life and death. Yes, like I said, we shall all die one day, but we have the responsibility to extend our lives just a little more, if we can.

So, eating plant-based food has been associated with lowering the probability of obesity and many chronic illnesses, like heart disease, type 2 diabetes (T2D), cancer and inflammation. Plant-based nutrition would include vegetables, fruits, legumes, seeds, whole grains, nuts and other products. This nutritional pattern is associated with a lower risk of suffering from several illnesses in our lives. The Whole Foods Plant Based Diet (WFPBD) is known to encourage a better and appropriate weight, better levels of cholesterol, blood glucose and less worries about blood pressure. Evidence is bound that with this state of affairs, one is less likely to take or depend on medication to treat these chronic complaints.

Another well researched advantage of plant-based food is the prevention and or indeed reversal of heart diseases, diabetes and slowing down of some types of cancer. Note here that the plant-based diets do not just work as preventative measures, that is to prevent many chronic illnesses, but they also work to reverse the illnesses in case someone already has them. Further, plant-based food is known to improve symptoms from chronic sicknesses such as inflammatory bowel disease, rheumatoid arthritis, gout and multiple sclerosis.

With the above in mind, it can be deduced, that plants remain powerful sources of numerous nutrients that are essential for excellent wellbeing and holistic health. Plants have vitamins, minerals, fibre, protein and good carbohydrates. Studies have exhibited that having a diet superior in plant foods and low in animal foods has been linked to a lower risk of chronic diseases, compared with people having a diet low in plant foods. This plant-based pattern focuses on the complete diet rather than single foods or supplementation, which T. Colin

Campbell and Thomas M. Campbell II, MD in *The China Study* and Prof. Michael Pollan's *In Defence of Food* refer to as *reductionism* and *nutritionism* respectively. It is argued that supplements are derived from real, whole foods. Why not, therefore, eat the whole foods which contain other important nutrients within it? Food has been reduced to its miniature components due to the business acumen. But there is no *substitute* for a diet that is healthy, which holistically has whole and real foods.

Scientific research shows that eating a diet high in vegetables and fruits and less refined and animal foods may bring down the number of people that suffer from chronic disease such as stroke, diabetes, high blood pressure, heart disease and cancer. ***In short, a plant-based nutrition cuts across all the diseases irrespective of their nature.*** Some researchers and nutritionists have recommended that individuals should not worry about devising or allocating specific foods or counting calories for specific aliments because plants have shown in many ways to address most of the many disease that affect us every day. A Whole Foods Plant Based Nutrition is known to have instantaneous health benefits by improving one's immunity, increasing energy levels, not forgetting improving one's complexion.

It is important, henceforth, to keep in mind that there is no need to go on a diet, because diets are a temporal measure and therefore, do not work. Fad diets are a quick fix. And so, it is easy come, easy go. You cannot make drastic changes just like that, because you have been used to eating in a certain way or pattern for many years. Such eating habits are hard to let go in a fad. So, just as much as your present situation or condition took long to resurface, you ought to expect that the remedy should equally not be a quick fix. The quicker you want to fix it, the more forceful it will come back, even being worse than before.

The most important thing to do is to eat right and the body will fix itself. I am also not calling on you to abandon what you are eating right now. Like I said, what you eat is your choice and health is a critical choice, but all am saying is that take a deep breath and you may wish to appreciate the other alternative at hand. You will be surprised to learn that there is a better life on the other side than what may be obtaining now, which has been taken as normal. It is better to make short tangible changes that will accumulatively give you the desired outcome and a permanent solution.

I remember some time ago; I watched a TV programme where Bill Cosby was chatting with kids (*You can watch it on YouTube*). The programme was about whether kids liked vegetables or not, on a programme called *Kids Say the Darndest Things - Have Some Veggies*. It was funny to watch though, but it sent me a message that kids nowadays have grown up not to like plant-based foods because of the booming processed food industry and the discretionary foods which their parents have made them get used to. They know snacks to be candy, biscuits, waffles, flakes, chips, chocolate and all manner of empty nutrients diary and animal processed products. I also remember one day telling my kids in a supermarket to buy what they wanted to eat. Their basket was filled up with processed foods and I did not blame them, but I had the responsibility to advise them on the merits and most importantly, demerits of such foods.

Critical Food Nutrients

Indispensable nutrients of food are those that our bodies cannot produce or cannot produce in adequate quantities. They are derived from food in order to promote growth, repair, prevent disease and enhance overall good health. People need not be obsessed with religiously categorising these foods and ensuring they are counting calories and their sources. There is no food which would contain all the nutrients because all the things we eat (especially a variety of vegetable and fruits, legumes, nuts and seeds), have a mixture of all these important things.

Nutrients come in two categories: *macronutrients* and *micronutrients*. As the name implies, we need macronutrients in *big* quantities and include the main content of the diet. These are Carbohydrates, Fats and Proteins. Minerals and Vitamins, (we can even add phytonutrients, antioxidants and or bioactives), are micronutrients and their *small* amounts are very critical for good health. Broadly speaking, almost all macronutrients supply us the energy we need and micronutrients assists the body to unlock and use the energy.

The fuel or energy source for our bodies and muscles is derived from carbohydrates. The brain and just all cells need energy. They are found in big amounts in potatoes, bread, grains, pasta, sugar and even in nuts, fruits and vegetables. Simple table sugar is equally a kind of carbohydrate. Protein is needed for repair and growth and does provide us with the building blocks, growth and repair for our bodies. We need 9 essential amino acids from protein. It is eminent in most animal foods like dairy, eggs, nuts, legumes and other foods like quinoa and other legumes. Fats are necessary for the over-all wellness and health. Fats have the highest level of energy as compared to the other two (Proteins and Carbohydrates have four (4) calories as equated to fats with nine (9) calories per gram, while alcohol has seven (7)). Fats can be found in nuts, meat, oil, fish, avocado,

So Why Plants?

There are several propositions about which diet is the ideal one for you. However, it is indisputable that nutrition and food that stresses real, whole, fresh produce and reduced refined foods are recommendable and significant for inclusive health and wellness. The Whole Foods Plant Based Nutrition does just that. This pays particular attention to less or unrefined foods, precisely plants and it is feasible in inspiring and maintaining good health.

No one would outrightly define what a plant-based nutrition is all about, because this is simply a way of life or a lifestyle and not *dieting* per say. The reason is nutrition that is plant-based may differ to a large extent grounded on the level to which one incorporates animal derived products in their food. People that adhere to this way of eating do eat mostly plants, but products from animals may or may not be part of their food. That said, the underlying premises of a Whole Foods Plant-Based Nutrition (WFPBN), among others, stresses that the food should be *unprocessed* or indeed slightly treated or refined.

At the same time, the products from animals should be limited or wholly avoided, because the main essence here should be the plant aspect of food that centres on fruits, vegetables, legumes, whole grains, nuts and seeds. This should constitute most of the stuff eaten. You can observe from the above that WFPBN, does not include highly processed foods such as white flour, vegetable oils milk products and the main culprit, sugar. On the whole, WFPBN pays particular consideration to the quality and source of the food. In this regard, *local farmers' market* is the ideal avenue for such food, where framers and others sell real, whole and possibly organic produce.

Whole Foods Plant-Based Nutrition has been seen to be good for the heart, weight control, environmental protection and generally, holistic health.

*   *   *

Science researchers may not reach a consensus on whether it is the fibre, the limited calories or the mighty antioxidants in the plants that put them at an upper hand for our health. Many studies and research indicate that a diet that is high in vegetables, fruits, wholegrains, legumes, nuts and seeds increases the longevity and reduces the incidence of chronic illnesses like cancer, obesity, stroke, diabetes and heart disease.

As human beings, science has showed that we are able to survive without meat and without carbohydrates (especially highly refined ones). But we cannot survive long enough without plants. Dr. Peter Brukner from Australia, a sports medicine doctor and founder of *SugarByHalf* further argues in his book, *A Fat Lot of Good*, that we can survive without carbohydrates, but we absolutely need fats and proteins.

Plants have all necessary micronutrients we need such as minerals, phytonutrients and vitamins that our cells badly need, aside from the macronutrients; the proteins, carbohydrates and fats. Of course, there is always the worry about vitamin B12, which is mostly inherent in animal foods like eggs, fish and meat. Plants are referred to as being nutrient-dense than any other food we can think of, comprising numerous biologically active elements that have a physiological impact on our cells. Various forms of carbs found in plants do act as prebiotics, that assist to grow healthy and good gut bacteria (probiotics) that help keep our immune system, thyroid and digestive tracts healthy. Some nuts, brown rice, onions and pulses all contribute as prebiotics.

Plants have Fibre

I mentioned earlier about Fibre. Dietary fibre is a type of carbohydrate or starch that is indigestible in the body. Fibre is plentiful in nuts, fruits, vegetables, cereals, grains and legumes among others. It can be soluble, insoluble and resistant. Dietary fibre has to work together to be effective. It is also a nutrient dense plant-based food and an important part of our health because of several reasons:

- Controls our blood sugar (Glucose). This delays the assimilation of glucose into the blood, significant for the management of diabetes.
- Controls or reduces cholesterol absorption by attaching to it in the gut.
- It helps with the bowel movements.
- It helps with our satiety, that is helps us feel fuller for longer and avoid overeating.
- Assists in the risk reduction of colorectal cancer, diabetes and heart disease.
- It contributes to the good health of the colon by feeding the healthy bacteria.
- It helps in retaining water that is sent back to the body systems in the process of homeostasis.
- Fibre also fends off many cravings for those highly refined or processed snacks.

Soluble fibre dissolves in water. It assists in slowing down the bowel discharge in the stomach, promoting satiety or making you and I feel fuller for longer. It also controls blood glucose and cholesterol levels. You can find this type of fibre in food like vegetables, fruits, barley, legumes and oats.

Insoluble fibre, however, doesn't get dissolved in water, but it is known to absorb water that helps to soften the stool and support normal and frequent bowel movements and keeping its environment healthy. It is vital therefore to improve your fluid consumption as you increase your fibre. With no fluid, the fibre remains tough, making it challenging to pass through and causing constipation. The fibre enables someone to pass normal and regular faeces. Ever wondered why some people that wholly eat highly processed foods and the reason why they don't go to the toilet? Some even boast that they go to the toilet only once in two or more days! Where does all the junk food they eat go? It is certainly right in the body somewhere, where its causing chaos and destruction. The recommended number of times to go to the toilet for bowel movements should be not less than two times in a day and the type or colour of the faeces does matter, reminiscent of the food that you ate earlier. One can find this type of fibre in seeds, nuts, skin of fruits, vegetables and wholegrain breads and cereals.

Resistant Fibre or *starch* does not get handled in the small intestine but goes to the big intestine or colon. Resistant starch (and some soluble fibre) work as prebiotics (which is like food) for probiotics (good bacteria) present in the large bowel that are critical for digestive health. Resistant starch can be obtained in cooked and cooled potato, under ripe bananas, undercooked pasta and rice. Resistant Starch can also come about in an event of heating up followed by cooling of certain foods like potato or rice. Food with lots of this starch usually has glycaemic index that is low.

Dietary fibre, whether soluble, insoluble or resistant, may not be found in isolation. It is usually found in a mixed set up, that is with other fibres. It is, therefore, critical to ensure that it is consumed in a manner that allows effectivity. If the different aspects of fibre are separated, it may not work successfully. For instance, resistant starch rarely is assessed when fibre is evaluated in a food and it might underestimate the amount of fibre in a particular food.

Note also that when you eat plant-based food, you promote the presence of good bacteria in the gut, that take the fibre we eat and make *short-chain fatty acids*, such as *Butyrate*. Butyrate protects us from cancer, especially colorectal cancer (colon and rectum cancer).

Because we feed these good bacteria with plant food, they pay us back by protecting us. If we don't feed them, the colon cancer cells may grow. Once the cancer cells are exposed to the concentration of butyrate that our good bacteria make in our gut when we eat fibre, the growth of the cancer cells is stopped. Therefore, eating plenty of fibre rich foods, especially from plants, will almost always shield off these cancer cells in the colon and rectum.

Foods that are rich in fibre include:

Vegetables

Vegetable that have a deep dark colour, generally have a higher content of fibre. These would include spinach, lettuce, carrots, beets, broccoli, potatoes and kale.

Fruits

The fruits that are rich in Fibre include mangoes, apples, bananas, oranges, and most berries.

Legumes and Beans

Beans and legumes are known to have a lot of good flavour and packed with fibre. These would include beans of all types, lentils and peas.

Nuts

May include almonds, pistachios, pumpkin seeds, sunflower seeds, groundnuts and others.

Plants have antioxidants and phytonutrients

Vegetables and fruits have special plant nutrients that neutralise a lot of the toxins that we take in. Kris Carr, in her book, *Crazy Sexy Diet,* refers to phytonutrients as *Secret Service Agents that protect and fight off diseases in plants.* Plants contain most of the phytonutrients (or phytochemicals) that have natural antioxidants which are polyphenolics occurring in all parts of the plant such as the stems, bark, wood, fruit, leaves, flowers, roots, seeds, pollen and seeds. They are in thousands. Phytonutrients come in all flavours and colours and this gives plants their variety characteristic colours like red, green, yellow, orange, pink and so on. The more the colours, the more present antioxidants are expected.

Antioxidant activities in the plants vary but may work as reducing agents and as free radical scavengers or acceptors among others. Too much acid in the body destabilises the body and puts too much pressure on the crucial body parts such as the liver and kidneys. In the process of neutralising the acids, some *guys* called *free radicals* are created which may be lethal to the cells. These molecules lose one of their electrons which make them unstable. To stabilise themselves, they need to grab an electron from another molecule and that molecule in turn becomes a free radical (some call them short form, *free rads*) and that creates a circus. In excess, these free rads can damage cells and can be carcinogenic.

The body manufactures these *antioxidants* whose main goal is to deal with free radicals. What happens is that antioxidants are known to be givers and so they do donate their extra electron to the avaricious free radicals which in turn stabilise. The antioxidant does this by delivering the electron through the liver and once it does that, it returns to the blood stream to check on the other free radicals and start the process all over again. And so, as many antioxidants as possible, will enable you control these *bad boys* time and again and prevent oxidative stress, aging and damage to the precious cells and ultimately prevent diseases such as some cancers. But, if you have too many of the free rads, the body gives up and your health starts a nosedive! Mind you, not all free rads are bad, others are good as they deal with foreign bodies and waste.

In this regard, when you eat phytonutrients found in plants, the corresponding positive effect equally benefits you. It is advisable to eat them raw because most of them can be affected by heating. However, some of them like lycopene and beta-carotene maybe more bioavailable once heated or semi processed.

There is a wide variety of antioxidants occurring naturally, that come in form of minerals, enzymes and vitamins among others. As minerals, this includes Zinc, Manganese, Selenium and Copper. Vitamins include A, C and E preventing peroxidation damage in the biological system. Enzymes are like superoxide dismutase and (SOD) and Glutathione Peroxidase (GPx).

Concrete examples of these include *lycopene* found in watermelons, tomatoes, pink grapefruits. These may help prevent prostate cancer. Others are Resveratrol found in grapes, blueberries and some red wine. There is also *beta-carotene* that comes from orange coloured plant foods like sweet potatoes, carrots and winter squash. The body converts beta-carotene into Vitamin A, which is good for our sight. Other antioxidants are *quercetin* which is found in onion and apples and known to prevent heart illness and another is *lutein* and *zeaxanthin* that is prevalent in corn and so on.

As you can see, antioxidants are really good for us, but they should not be isolated and packed into a capsules or pills called *supplements*. Most of these supplements are of very poor quality and may not contain the actual nutrients or may contain too much of the nutrient. Most of them, therefore, don't work. A diet that is balanced and that includes an extensive assortment of colourful vegetables and fruits is what actually works. Eat more plants than anything else and reduce the meat products and you will be doing your body a tremendous act of kindness.

Phytonutrients are present in most coloured vegetables and fruits, beans, grains and other plants. Others can be found in resveratrol in red wine (though still be cognisant that wine is acidic, you are better off eating real red berries or grapes), polyphenols found in tea, cruciferous vegetables (cabbage family of broccoli, kale, cauliflower, bok choy, brussels sprouts, collards, kohlrabi, turnip greens and mustard greens), have isothiocyanates.

Plants have Minerals and Vitamins

Minerals found in water and soil effortlessly find their route into the body all through the animal and plant food we eat. This could be fish or liquids consumed. But it is harder to move vitamins from the food and from elsewhere into our bodies because cooking and storage and sheer exposure of these vitamins to air can deactivate these more delicate compounds.

Minerals

If you go to a supermarket, you will be bombarded by so many food stuffs in the middle aisles announcing and inviting you to buy them because they have a rich content of minerals and vitamins. Most of these foods talk to you and they are packaged in bright colours to attract you. However, we rarely think of minerals and vitamins as that important, but hey, these micronutrients are super. Some of them are in animal products like meat (with iron) and milk (with calcium), but most of them are in plants.

Minerals are said to be inorganic and exist with their biochemical composition. They assist the body develop, grow and remain healthy. The body utilises various minerals to carry out various roles like developing bones that are strong and conveying nerve impulses. Other minerals can be used to produce hormones or the maintenance of a regular heartbeat.

Two kinds of minerals do exist and that is *macro* and *trace*. *Macro* implies big amount as the body requires bigger amounts of some minerals. These may include potassium, phosphorus, calcium, magnesium, sodium, sulphur and chloride. The smaller amounts or trace, needed in smaller quantities by the body could be iodine, zinc, fluoride, manganese, copper, selenium and cobalt.

Our bodies require and store, relatively substantial amounts of major minerals. Among the core responsibilities of main minerals is to sustain the appropriate *equilibrium of water in our bodies*. Potassium, chloride and sodium are in the forefront for such tasks. The three other main minerals; magnesium, calcium and phosphorus, are vital for strong bones. Sulphur assists in stabilising structures of protein, with some of those that make up nails, skin and hair.

Note that an overabundance of one mineral may affect the availability of the other. These sorts of disparities are typically instigated by excesses from food additions or supplements, and not real food sources. For instance, calcium attaches with surplus sodium and is expelled when the body detects that levels of sodium must be reduced. This means that if you consume too much sodium out of table salt or highly processed foods, you may end up losing the required calcium as the body clears itself of the excess sodium. Likewise, excessive phosphorus can deter our capabilities to assimilate magnesium.

The trace minerals (micro minerals) do many things such as iron transporting oxygen in the entire body, zinc helping in blood clotting and vital for smell and taste and strengthening the immune response, while copper assisting in making several enzymes. Other minerals assist in preventing injury to cells of the body and being part of key enzymes or augmenting their activity. Examples of these trace minerals are chromium, fluoride, iodine, molybdenum and selenium. A slight surplus of manganese may aggravate deficiency of iron whilst too little may also cause issues. When we have very small amount of iodine, the thyroid hormone production reduces, causing lethargy and weight increase as well as other physical conditions. The crisis worsens if the body also has too little selenium.

Just to highlight the need for a few minerals such as:

Iron

The body requires iron to carry oxygen from the lungs to the entire body. The body requires oxygen to live and stay healthy. Iron is critical in the production of Haemoglobin, which is a component of red blood cells carrying oxygen all over the body. Leafy green vegetables, like broccoli and baked potato skin are some of the plant foods rich in Iron. Others are beans, kale, pumpkin seeds, quinoa, chia seeds, lentils, tofu, cashew nuts and so on.

Potassium

Potassium maintains the nervous system and the muscles in optimal working condition. Plant foods rich in it are potatoes, tomatoes, sweet potatoes with skin on, bananas and green vegetables such as broccoli, spinach and fruits like oranges, and legumes such as beans, lentils and split peas. Potassium is rapidly assimilated into the blood, where it spreads easily and the kidneys expel it, much like a water-soluble vitamin.

Zinc

Zinc assists the immune system, which is the body's system to fight infections and illnesses. It also assists with growth of cells and assists to heal wounds, like cuts. Nuts like cashews, almonds, peanuts and legumes such as beans, lentils and split peas do contain zinc.

*   *   *

When individuals do not have adequate amounts of these vital minerals, they may develop health challenges. For example, not enough calcium, in particular when you are a kid, may lead to bones that are weak. You may take mineral supplements, but most people and children don't require them if they have a healthful diet. Phosphorus, potassium, calcium and magnesium and so on, are all essential for our cells and they do participate in cell signalling. So, it is important to consume those minerals and remain healthy!

Vitamins

As micronutrients, the vitamins are classified as *organic* and air, acid and heat could break them down. They are as critical as minerals because of their hundreds of roles in our bodies. Enough of vitamins is necessary but at the same time avoid an excess that may be toxic. A healthy diet is still the finest means to get adequate or appropriate amounts of vitamins.

Every day, our bodies produce skin, bone and muscles. Red blood with oxygen and important nutrients get to all areas of the body and nerve signals are sent throughout our bodies and come up with chemical signals that move from one organ to another, delivering directives that assist to maintain life. The body, therefore, needs some special supply of resources that includes at least 30 vitamins, minerals and vitalities. The body requires these but cannot adequately make them itself.

Vitamins are deemed nutrients that are necessary, due to the fact that they accomplish hundreds of functions in our body like wound recovery, strengthening of the immune system, bone health, cell damage repair and energy production from food. They are needed in small amounts, hence the term micronutrients. But the inability to get those miniature amounts can spell doom for your health. Some vitamins are fat-soluble like A, D, E and K. They can also be water soluble like the B complex and C.

For instance, we need vitamin C to prevent diseases like scurvy or gum bleeding. We need vitamin A to prevent blindness. Vitamin D is important among other things to prevent rickets caused by fragile bones that bring about distortions in skeleton like curved legs. A mix of appropriate phosphorus, vitamin K & D, magnesium and calcium, can safeguard us from bone fissures. For pregnant mothers, they are encouraged to take Folic acid or Folate to prevent birth defects such as brain and spinal flaws in children.

Micronutrients work interdependently. Take for example vitamin C. This vitamin helps in the absorption of iron. On the other hand, vitamin D lets our bodies obtain calcium from sources of food traversing the gastrointestinal area instead of plucking it from the bones. The micronutrient interchange is nevertheless not always supportive: vitamin C bars our bodies' aptitude to integrate copper, which is a vital mineral. Research shows that even a slight excess in manganese mineral would deteriorate the iron deficit.

It is the watery sections of the food we eat where water-soluble vitamins are loaded. They are grasped immediately into the blood as food is digested or during the dissolution of supplements. Due to the fact that the body consist of more than 60% water, several of the water-soluble vitamins go around the body without challenges. Kidneys endlessly control the levels of these vitamins and releasing surplus ones out in the urine. Vitamin C and B are Water soluble vitamins. The latter constitutes B1 or *Thiamine*, B2 or *Riboflavin*, B3 or *Niacin*, B5 or *Pantothenic acid*, B9 or *Folic acid* and B12 or *Cobalamin*.

Despite several functions, among their most significant function is assisting to grab the energy in the food that we eat. Most tissues in the body are kept healthy because of these vitamins. Further, vitamins maintain health in many ways; for instance, B vitamins are essential elements of some coenzymes in distributing energy from the food. Riboflavin, niacin, thiamine and pantothenic acid take part in production of energy while vitamins B12, folic acid and B6 work on amino acids and assist in the multiplication of cells. Some key tasks of vitamin C are to assist make collagen, which weaves together abrasions, helps the walls of the blood vessels and creates a foundation for bones and teeth.

Research has shown that certain water-soluble vitamins may remain in the body for a long time and one may have many years of quantities of say, vitamin B12, which the liver stores. Similarly, vitamin C and folic acid stores are known to stay on for at least two days. But because of the nature of the vitamins, they have to be replaced daily or every few days. Keep in mind that consumed in excess, vitamins can be toxic, especially through supplements. For instance, exceptionally elevated amounts of B6 may harm nerves, instigating muscle weakness and numbness.

Fat-soluble vitamins enter the blood via lymph networks in the stomach walls. Several of the fat-soluble vitamins move in the body under the guide of proteins which act as carriers. Foods with fat and oils have fat-soluble vitamins. In the body, the liver and fat tissues behave as the major sticking regions for vitamins and circulate when required. During absorption of food in the body, fat-soluble vitamins move into the lymph vessels prior to getting into the bloodstream. Usually, a protein accompanies these vitamins in order to go around the body.

Throughout the body, these vitamins are utilised and fat tissues and the liver store the surplus. If there is need for additional amounts, the body gets from the reservoir, freeing them from the liver to the bloodstream.

Fat-soluble vitamins maintain your eyes, nervous system, lungs, gastrointestinal tract and skin in good repair. It would be difficult to form bones without such vitamins as D, A and K. Our eyes are also protected by keeping the cells healthy. Vitamin E helps in absorption and storage of vitamin A while Vitamin E equally functions as an antioxidant that helps shield the body against free radicals. Because the body stores fat-soluble vitamins for long, toxic levels may pile up which would take place if you, for example, consume supplements. It is very uncommon for whole, real food to bring about too much of a vitamin.

A word on Vitamin D and B12

Vitamin D

Vitamin D is among several nutrients the body needs to be healthy. It is considered both a nutrient that we can take in and also considered as a hormone that the body makes. Very limited foods could be naturally rich in vitamin D, (that is the reason why most people turn to supplementation); so, the main nutritional source of this vitamin, are foods that are fortified and supplements. Some sources are breakfast cereals and dairy products (both are vitamin D fortified), and fatty fish like tuna and salmon. The body produces vitamin D from cholesterol, through a method triggered by sunlight on our skin, that is why it is called the *sunshine vitamin*. Darker skinned toned people do not make enough Vitamin D through this process, just like older, overweight and when you cover yourself up while in the sun. Studies show that mushrooms that are grown in direct sunlight, have in them Vitamin D. In this regard, mushrooms from the wild or naturally grown in the bush ought to have high levels of Vitamin D. For commercial or domestic grown ones, it is believed that once they are exposed to enough sunlight, they are able to accumulate Vitamin D.

Vitamin D assists to retain and absorb calcium and phosphorus, which are crucial for the building of bones. It assists in absorbing calcium, that eventually makes bones and keeps them healthy. Severe decreased vitamin D levels can result in brittle and soft bones as well as muscle weakness and pain. Studies show that several organs of the body and tissues have vitamin D receptors and many research studies associate low levels of vitamin D to osteoporosis or bone fractures in adults. It could also function in the muscle and immune system.

When our skin is exposed to the sun, Vitamin D is produced. The amount produced in this manner depends on factors like the time of the year or season, time of the day, the extent of cloud cover, pollution of the air and place where you stay. The Ultraviolet rays of the sun triggers the production of vitamin D in the skin. Deficiency is therefore common in areas with minimal amounts of everyday sunlight.

The metabolism of vitamin D is a complicated process. Because it is a fat-soluble vitamin, excess amounts can be stored in fat tissues and other tissues. Studies indicate that it is difficult to establish how long a daily dose of vitamin D would stay in the body, but it seems that big quantities will last for roughly ***two months***. In order to meet the requirement of vitamin D for the body, it is advisable to consume plenty health food from the entire food classes and get exposed to the sun appropriately.

Vitamin B12

Vitamin B12 (*Cobalamins)* is a water-soluble vitamin. It is a critical vitamin because it is required for health of the nerve tissue, function of the brain, red blood cell production and assisting in the creation and regulation of DNA. It influences the exterior and bone marrow, skin, central nervous systems, bones, vessels and mucous membranes as well as the regular growth of infants. Low levels of the vitamin can lead to irretrievable neurological disorders.

Because it is water soluble, it is capable of dissolving in water and go around the bloodstream. Research shows that our bodies can store B12 between **three** to **five years**. Any extra or undesirable vitamin B12 is expelled in the urine.

Cell metabolism in the body depends on vitamin B12, because it performs an essential role in fatty acid synthesis and production of energy. It allows for the energy discharge by supporting the body with folic acid absorption. Millions of red blood cells are produced by our bodies every minute and the cells would not reproduce appropriately in the absence of vitamin B12. The production of red blood cells declines if vitamin B12 is not balanced. Disorders like anaemia may take place if the count of red blood cell comes down.

In nature, vitamin B12 is in animal products, like meat, fish, dairy products and eggs. It does not normally exist in plant foods, that's why debate rages as to why vegans may be at risk without supplementation. Necessary it is at all times to have a balanced diet and derive adequate nutrient quantities.

The bottom line is that vitamins and minerals are wholly useful in the body if they are derived from whole and real foods other than supplements. The use of supplements should not be in excess and should be through the guidance of a physician. Supplements should also be of high degree of quality for them to be useful.

Some food sources of vitamins and minerals:
Fat-soluble

Vitamin A: sweet potatoes, pumpkins carrots, spinach, mangoes.

Vitamin D: sun-grown mushrooms, sunlight itself, some cereal, fatty fish.

Vitamin E: whole grains, leafy green vegetables, nuts.

Vitamin K: eggs, cabbage, milk, kale, spinach, broccoli.

Water-soluble

B-1: acorn squash, watermelon.

B-2: whole and enriched grains.

B-3: mushrooms, whole grains, potatoes.

B-5: mushrooms, whole grains, broccoli, avocados.

B-6: bananas, legumes, soy foods (e.g. tofu).

B-7: some fish, whole grains.

B-9: broccoli, asparagus, spinach, legumes (black-eyed peas and chickpeas).

B-12: fortified soymilk and cereals, some meat, poultry, fish.

Vitamin C: broccoli, citrus fruit, potatoes, bell peppers, spinach, strawberries, tomatoes, brussels sprouts.

Major minerals

Calcium: leafy green vegetables, salmon.

Chloride: salt

Magnesium: broccoli, spinach, legumes, seeds, whole-wheat bread.

Potassium: vegetables, fruits, grains, legumes.

Sodium: vegetables, salt, soy sauce.

Trace minerals

Chromium: nuts, some poultry, some fish.

Copper: nuts, seeds, whole-grain products, beans, prunes, shellfish.

Fluoride: fish, teas.

Iodine: iodized salt, seafood.

Iron: fruits, green vegetables, eggs, some meat, poultry.

Manganese: nuts, legumes, whole grains, tea.
Selenium: some seafood, walnuts.
Zinc: whole grains, legumes, some shellfish.

*   *   *

Enough of vitamins and minerals. Let's get back to the catalogue and importance of plant-based food.

Plants have low sugar content

As a matter of importance, real, whole food is lower in sugar than many highly processed foods. Despite fruit containing sugar, it is nevertheless also high in water, vitamins, minerals and fibre, making it much healthier than soda and processed foods. A whole foods plant-based nutrition could also help reduce cravings for sweet things like biscuits, candy and cakes. Once the body adjusts to eating whole real, unrefined or unprocessed foods, cravings for sugary foods tremendously reduce and would subsequently vanish because the taste buds will ultimately adjust to welcome real food within a given period of time (nutritionist say within 6 months).

Plant food is environmentally and animal friendly

The world population has kept growing; and so, more food is required and will be required to feed the people. To supply food to this growing population, presents an environmental strain due to deforestation, fuel needs, use of pesticides, industrial packaging and greenhouse emissions. Creating ecological agriculture premised on real, whole food could help enhance planet health by decreasing energy needs and lessening the quantities of non-biodegradable garbage that people produce. Agriculture is known to account for more than 65% of freshwater use, becoming the planet's biggest water-guzzling area. So, to produce dairy and meat products, it is estimated that you need massive amounts of water. Studies show that growing crops uses less water than producing meat and dairy products. Therefore, more plant food may save more water. Further, plant food may also promote animal life, for those that advocate for animal rights and for religious reasons.

Plant food is good for Immunity

Human beings have powerful immune systems which would only work optimally if one eats more plants. Dr. Joel Fuhrman, in his book, *Super Immunity,* says that 70% of the immune system is located in the gastrointestinal tract and the bacterial population of this area makes up a complex ecosystem that can be seen as an organ of the body. Dr. Fuhrman adds that when we eat a healthy, nutrient dense plant-based food, we encourage the development of the good microorganisms which play a critical role in strengthening our immunity.

When we are exposed to harmful elements, the immune system kicks into action, with defense against infectious organisms and other invaders. The specialised cells of a strong immune system, proteins, tissues and organs continuously monitor what is in our bodies and respond when needed.

A healthy immune function begins with what we eat. Plant foods positively appear to be anti-inflammatory, antioxidant, anti-angiogenesis and anticancer. In this case, eating more vegetables, fruits, whole grains, legumes and nuts is a substantial characteristic of excellent immune function. Further, many scientific findings have connected obesity with a diminished immune reaction and therefore, a plant-based approach may address that challenge. A well-balanced diet that has immune-boosting plant-based foods found in vegetables and fruits are nutrient dense, containing important nutrients like potassium that helps lower blood pressure, antioxidants that have shown to fight most cancers and enhance the optimal health of the brain.

Plants are less expensive

Most times, people would comment and argue that organic and real, whole food is expensive than highly refined food. Just as much as it may be true, the difference is minimal if one equates this to the astronomical cost that comes with nursing chronic illnesses, a cost which is not only individual, but also governmental. Because of the chronic nature of the diseases, one spends more money for a long time just as the Government's healthcare system does. It would be better, therefore, to spend less money on buying real, whole and unprocessed food. Whole food costs less in the long term, because the chances are very high that it will most certainly promote you to live healthier, happier and longer.

Plant Food has no health claims

As noted earlier, highly processed food in the middle aisles of the supermarket has so much health claims, statements made by the food industries during advertising and on food labels. On the other hand, fresh plant food which is real whole food in the fresh food section, does not claim anything because everyone knows that this food is already healthy food.

Plants offer a high degree of authenticity

How many times have you watched videos, watched on the news or read in newspapers and magazines, online social media about fake meat products produced in backyards; meat purported to be human flesh, sausage or polony suspected to be something else and some food made from plastics and so many other stories! This tells you why you should trust plants. Even though it could be infested with some chemicals, at least you can see and taste that it is a plant. You will also not be deterred by plant food being organic because to a large extent, you still get a reasonable amount of nutrients from it, than junk, highly processed or meat imitations which are vastly detrimental to your cells and to your health.

Plant food slows aging

Dr. Michael Greger, founder of *Nutritionfacts.org*, in his book, *How Not to Die,* says *telomeres* are seen as the *life fuse* because they may begin diminishing as soon as we are born and when they are gone, we are dead too.

Certain things are a given in life, like aging, but understanding why we get old or the cause of aging, is a conundrum that scientists are still battling with. Some scientists think we have to blame too much sugar consumption, others think it is oxidative stress wreaking havoc on our DNA, it is chronic inflammation or indeed we are simply in tune with what we are supposed to go through. However, a theory that stands out prominently is that we have these tiny caps called *telomeres,* located at the tip of each of our chromosomes, that are small shielding tops at the ends of the DNA molecules. Their job is to stop the ends of chromosomes from wearing out or sticking to each other. They comprise an identical arrangement of six (6) nucleotides recurring over and over again and the recurrence brings about disposability. At any point when the cells divide, part of the cap vanishes and when it completely vanishes, cells would die. Studies show that scientists can take some DNA from the blood and estimate how old an individual was in as far as the length of the telomeres is concerned.

Dr. Greger argues that we can prevent the cap of the telomere from vanishing by, for example, stopping to smoke as well as minding the food we eat. He states that the eating of vegetables and fruits, which are packed with phytonutrients, is linked with longer protective telomeres and a longer, healthier life.

Plants help our Genes and DNA

Genes express in a certain way. The *expression* denotes the procedure where information from a gene's DNA system is interpreted into something like a protein, which in turn is used in the structure of the cell or function. Studies show that nearly all our genes and DNA could be affected by our diet that consequently affects our body systems. Our genes are known to impact on our metabolism processes, but they are only able to express well if they are given the right environment, such as food. That is the reason why the food that parents and grandparents ate, is seen to manifest in the offsprings because scientists believe that diet can vary the make-up of one's DNA and the changes passed on to posterity. So, with the foregoing in mind, the more appropriate the food we eat, the better the gene expression and this appropriate food is none other than plant-based.

Plants are good for the Microbiome

Microbiome is a set of bacteria that lives in the Gut and elsewhere in the body numbering in trillions. Their cells are said to outnumber our own by an average factor of 10 to 1. Adhering to whole food plant-based nutrition is known to be beneficial for this microbiome that promotes a healthy immune system, digestion, thyroid health and many more. It is also evident that several whole or real foods play a critical role as prebiotics, that in fact is food for the gut bacteria, fermented to form short-chain fatty acids. Additionally, to promote good gut health, these fatty acids could also enhance glucose metabolism.

Plant food promotes good teeth and skin

Everyone would love to have healthy teeth and that is what exactly plant food does. Highly refined carbohydrates and sugar stimulate dental degeneration (caries) by supplying the plaque-triggering microorganisms that reside in our mouths. The blend of acid and sugar in carbonated drinks is exceptionally expected to bring about this decay. Plant food does increase and balances the pH of the body and the good health of the teeth. For instance, white, green and black tea contribute in the protection of the teeth.

Studies show that plant-based nutrition also improves the skin and acne conditions. It has been observed that most people that eat more plants have less pimples and better complexion, because the natural phytonutrients in plants seemingly impact positively on the good texture of the skin. Studies and researchers have further revealed that most phytochemicals from plants neutralise free radicals that do aid aging. Fruit and vegetables have a range of vitamins like E and C that are potent antioxidants that counter free radicals and avoid development of wrinkles. The antioxidants equally decrease or inhibit chronic or long-term inflammation and assist collagen generation, making the skin more elastic. A plant-based nutrition increases the flow of blood in our bodies opening up arteries by dissolving plaque. Once blood flow is increased, this is for the good of the skin that now gets major vital nutrients, keeping it healthy and rejuvenated.

Plant food supports local produce

There are many farmers in the community that work hard to grow fresh produce. Most of these, especially, small scale farmers, do not use expensive chemicals such as fertilisers and pesticides to grow the produce. And so, apart from supporting and empowering these local farmers, you will also be buying produce that is near-organic, if not organic itself or indeed just fresh produce per excellence. Most of their produce such as vegetables, fruits grains, legumes, some dairy and some meat is not engulfed with harmful substances that may harm your cells. Their produce generally is cheaper than most chain supermarkets. They may sell this produce by the roadside or indeed, on a designated day and place. Such food is also very tasty and flavoury. Buy in bulk in advance.

Bottom line:

As you augment your personal health and wellness, consumption of real, whole foods may assist people that you care for to live healthy. Motivating family members and friends will be pronounced if you lead by example in assuming healthier eating behaviours. It is equally a decent approach to help children acquire knowledge about good nutrition at an early age.

Fad diets do not work. They easy come and they easy go. The mindset may be destructive as it restricts your concentration on your holistic and long-term sustainable health. Afterall, nutrition that is great is beyond just weight loss, which most people concentrate on. It is also about having sufficient liveliness and feeling healthier and happier longer.

Focusing on whole foods plant-based nutrition instead of dieting is a sure and viable and pleasant way of life. Instead of pushing loss of weight, let the weight be managed naturally due to the appropriate diet. I also like to encourage people to eat plant based food in the manner they had been eating junk food, *religiously.*

Whole foods plant-based nutrition is, but one element of a healthy living. It is also important to avoid a sedentary life and instead get plenty of exercise; avoid unnecessary stress, avoid toxins, get plenty of sleep, avoid unnecessary drugs and maintain a proper nutrition devoid of sugar, too much salt, vegetable oils, white flour and too much dairy. Eating whole foods and real foods that are plants, is one sure way of enhancing your health, guaranteeing your longevity and happy life.

The main message here to desirable health outcome, is to eat more fruits, vegetables, nuts, seeds, grains, legumes and other foods rich in nutrients. Eating highly processed food and excess inappropriate animal protein is detrimental to health. Avoid counting of calories and controlling the portion of food you eat. It is not necessary. Again, the way you eat junk now, should be the way you should be eating more plants. Even if you are overweight, the more plant food you eat, the more you will shade off excess weight and the better your health will become.

Here is a simple guidance that you may wish to consider. Remember to **Eat;**

- at least three (3) fruits per day.
- enough portions of salads and raw or partially cooked vegetables, daily.
- some nuts and seeds, preferably raw, per day.
- some beans and other legumes, daily.

*As much as possible, **Avoid** these noxious foods:*

- table sugar and other products with added sugar, like soft drinks (soda, fizzy drinks), biscuits, juices, cakes…
- vegetable oils, trans fats and margarine.
- most dairy products.
- deep fried foods, like chicken and chips.
- white flour and its associated products.
- braaied and highly refined or processed meat.
- foods with excess salt

With the above in mind, be cognisant with the food that you eat. When you go to buy food at the supermarket or grocery store, buy your food from the perimeter of the store, instead of the middle aisles, which have too many food claims and highly processed food. However, in an event that you still buy some highly processed food, develop the habit of checking the food labels and nutrition facts on the packaged foods. The ingredients and additives should not be too many and should not be difficult to pronounce. Google some of the additives if you can with your phone there and then.

If you decide to eat out at a restaurant, many food outlets do offer a variety of healthy choices now. Try and request for these or else stick with cooking at home. The more you cook your own meals, the more you know what you put; the quality and the quantity. Cooking and eating at home are also an important aspect as they bring families together and also encourages family members (especially the young) to embrace cooking as an important aspect of health. In this regard, you can eat anything, as long as you should cook or prepare it yourself.

EXERCISE, SLEEP & STRESS

Exercise

Exercise is important because it augments your good health. It can decrease your danger of chances of suffering from non-communicable diseases like diabetes, stroke and heart disease. Being physically active promotes both long- and short-term positive effects on your health. Significantly, frequent and steady exercise will, to a large extent, keep you well and live longer. Studies and researchers do recommend that on average, we should exercise at least 150 minutes in a week, or at a minimum of 30 minutes of bodily action in a day.

Exercise may not provide all the good effects of health if the aspect of food is ignored as stated earlier. However, it is one of the best things one can do, better than going on a diet. But do not expect to lose that much weight because of it. Take note that when you engage in physical activity, you are building the muscles and strengthening the bones, which is good for health, but it does not work to decrease your weight. That is why, if one is constant in having appropriate food and then adds physical activity or exercise on the equation, be assured that some reasonable weight will be lost. It explains why most physical trainers will also recommend that you have a *diet plan* because they know that exercise alone is not holistic.

Studies have also shown that more exercise can also help people with diabetes by improving insulin sensitivity due to the fact that it will build muscle unlike promotion of visceral body fat deposition. Exercise has also shown that the more you do it, the more you reduce depression, anxiety, fatigue, stress and elevated blood pressure. This is accomplished by the release of *feel good hormones* called *endorphins* as opposed to stress inducing hormone, *cortisol*.

Exercising triggers the body to preserve homeostasis by transmitting *lactate* to the muscles giving them energy. With time, this also indicates to the brain that it is time to stop physical exercise, in order for the muscles to get the needed oxygen. It brings about sweating, heavy breathing and the heart thumping. These traits are vital to the body in sustaining homeostasis. It affects oxygen levels, the body temperature, hydration and sugar levels, crucial for survival. The body utilises an automated response method to maintain normal water and temperature levels, to carry on the exercise. It is important to eat appropriately and drink enough liquids to assist retain homeostasis.

While exercising, the body requires to sustain a continuous amount of oxygen in the cells to assist the muscles at work, which may require additional oxygen than when they are at rest.

Do not bother about what kind of exercise. Do any exercise that makes you happy and that motivates you to do it. You should just sweat it out! There is no one exercise that fits all, never! We are all different and what works for one person may not work for the other. Consider small but significant changes from your day to day activities like cycling, walking instead of using your car, taking stairs instead of elevator or escalator, dancing or indeed jogging. For instance, park your car a little away from the place you are going to, so that you take advantage of the distance and time to walk. Don't spend more than an hour watching

TV without standing up and stretching. TV is considered an *obesogenic factor*, that is tending to promote obesity due to its sedentary nature.

Sleep

Sleep is a necessity just like drinking, eating and breathing. It adds holistically to the good health of someone and lack of it can bring about mental and physical drawbacks that include lack of concentration and productivity. It is categorised as non- Rapid Eye Movement and Rapid Eye Movement (REM). Non-REM sleep can be considered as gradual wave sleep or deep sleep, while when you are dreaming, it is REM sleep. But the point is the two patterns of sleep take place in a 3–5 cycles per night.

Getting adequate sleep will signal your capability to function properly during times you are not sleeping and enough good sleep at appropriate periods is good for your quality of life, mental health, safety and physical health. An inner body clock that regulates the time you are awake and when you are about to sleep, which follows the 24-hour repeat rhythm, is called the *circadian rhythm*. All cells, tissues and organs in the body are affected by this rhythm. Getting little sleep and not sleeping at appropriate times with poor type of sleep, makes you feel fatigue during the times you are awake, because you won't feel alert and refreshed. You may have issues with learning, focusing, remembering, driving, emotions, frustrations and so on. Not having enough sleep has also been associated with suicide and depression.

The *circadian rhythm* has two processes that work together to regulate the rhythm. Firstly, is the tension to slumber that intensifies with every moment you are wide awake that gets to a peak in the evening, time when most people fall asleep. Secondly, is the process concerning the inner clock of the body, which is in tandem with certain signals in the environment, like darkness and light that help control the awareness and sleepiness. Some light signals obtained through your eyes will signal a particular area in the brain that it is daylight, which area assist to associate the body clock with times of the day and night. The body releases *melatonin hormone* when it gets dark that signals to the body that it is time to get ready for bed and it helps you feel sleepy. The melatonin amount in the bloodstream is high as it gets to evenings and studies show that this is vital for preparing the body to get to sleep. Therefore, bright artificial light exposure from TV, computer, in the late evening may disrupt the process, becoming hard to fall asleep.

Sleep therefore is imperative as it helps how well the brain works. While asleep, the brain prepares for the next day and forms new trails to help with learning and memory. Therefore, a good night's sleep may help with learning as it helps someone in creativity, decision making, behaving well towards others and paying attention.

As you sleep, the body has the opportunity to build, repair and heal blood vessels which reduces the risk of chronic diseases. It also helps preserve a beneficial equilibrium of the *hormone, leptin* that makes you feel full and the *hormone, ghrelin* that makes you feel hungry. With inadequate sleep, ghrelin levels go up and leptin goes down, which will ultimately make you feel more hunger than before. Insulin is equally affected due to inadequate sleep as glucose levels rise, exacerbating diabetes risk. Chronic lack of sleep can also affect your body's immune system response to pathogens.

According to age, it is recommended that getting enough sleep could be between 12-16 hours a day for ages 4-12 months; 11-14 hours of sleep for 1-2 year olds; 10-13 hours of sleep for those aged 3-5; 9-12 hours for those aged 6-12; 8-10 hours for those for the 13-18 years and 7-8 hours if you are 18 years and above.

Stress
(Researched and written by Towela D. Banda)

In as far as the Australian Psychological Society is concerned, stress is feeling overwhelmed, usually occurring when faced with a situation that we feel we cannot handle. It is how the body responds to demands or threats which can either be real or imagined. We may experience some form of stress sometimes daily; that is just our body responding to what is threatening it. Stressors are circumstances that cause strain and may vary from person to person. A situation or circumstance that stresses one person may not stress the other, because each person has a different way of perceiving things. For example, the birth of a child can be stressful for one person and stress-free for another.

The common factors of stress include, work, school, relationship problems, financial difficulties, family, death of a loved one, illness or injury, marriage, divorce, job loss, intense traffic, gender identity crisis and retirement. Stress also has causes which are internal such as negative self-talk, self-doubt, need to always be perfect and having unrealistic expectations. It has symptoms which include headaches, sleep disorders, high blood pressure, fatigue, muscle tension, waking feeling tired, crying and poor memory.

Though it is usually referred to as *a negative,* it is not all stress that is bad. Some stressful situations can motivate us to finish tasks or push us to perform well. For example, during an examination when you see how little time you have to answer so many questions you are spurred into thinking or writing as fast as you can so that you are able to answer as many questions as possible; or when you hear a fire alarm in your apartment building, that swift response of quickly going outside and putting yourself out of danger, is also stress.

There are mainly two types of stress: *Chronic* and *Acute stress*. Acute stress lasts for a short period of time. Chronic stress on the other hand, goes on for a long time. It is Chronic stress that usually has effects on our health. These effects include depression, heart disease, diabetes, obesity, high blood pressure and sleep disorder. Studies show that stress levels rise and stay high usually when a person is encountering stressors continuously or has not had the opportunity to recover from the stressing situations or circumstances. Examples of such may include soldiers deployed to the war zone, who do not have time to recover from the stress of war because they are continuously in the environment that is causing them stress.

Knowing and trying to avoid our stressors is very important because stress if not managed, has negative effects on our health and overall wellbeing. If stress is ongoing for a long time, its effects can have a negative impact on our health both physically and mentally. Stress causes our bodies to produce high amounts of the stress hormones, *cortisol* and *adrenaline*. These hormones cause our heart rate to speed up and our blood pressure to rise up. This happens as part of what is known as *fight- or -flight* response, when our bodies prepare to face a challenging situation usually within a short period of time. The stress hormones circulate in our body system and keep us heightened. When these hormones reach a certain level, instead of helping us cope with stress, they have an opposite effect; they reduce the body's ability to handle stressful situations. Cortisol being one of the hormones that is released in excess by the body when we are stressed, is responsible for managing energy use and storage of fat in the body. *Cortisol is also known to encourage food cravings and increase appetite. Therefore, when we are stressed, our appetite increases, making us eat more. The more frequently we are stressed, the more we are likely to eat more, which leads to obesity.*

The more stressed a person is, the higher the chance of having heart diseases in comparison to those who are less stressed. This is because when a person is stressed the heart rate and blood pressure go up. So, one key effect of stress is *high blood pressure*. Apart from that, stress is known to contribute to other illnesses including cancer, irritable bowel syndrome and glandular problems and almost all psychological disorders, come as a result of stress. It also affects our memory because high levels of the hormone cortisol interfere with the human memory. When a person is stressed for less than six months, the effects on memory will not be permanent. However, long-term stress or chronic stress causes part of the brain where memory is stored to shrink. This means that if a person experiences stress for a long period of time, they are likely to suffer memory loss because the part of the brain where memory is stored would have shrunk.

Research and studies also show that depression is one of the outcomes or effects of stress, because it has been observed that the levels of the hormone cortisol are high in people with depression. The link between stress and depression is that cortisol decreases serotonin, (a hormone known to control the wellbeing and happiness). So, low serotonin causes depression. Toussaint, Dorn, Slavich and Shields (2014) carried out a research to determine how stress affected the physical and mental health of individuals. Their research found that there was a connection between poor mental health, physical health and stress. They also found that stressors like a loved one dying, pressure of school, financial problems and relationship difficulties, had a bad effect on mental and physical health of an individual, bringing about anxiety and depression.

A survey carried out on first year students at a college in South Africa found that about one in six students suffered from depression due to some experience during their childhood. Experiences such as being bullied, suffering emotional abuse or being neglected as children, were the major reasons that led to depression. The survey also found that apart from early childhood experiences, stressors that students had faced recently, such as unfaithful partners, break ups and gender identity crisis, also contributed to depression. It means, therefore, that stress, whether it happened in the past or recently, has a negative effect on our health. It does not only affect our physical or mental health when we are going through it but continues to have effects on our health long after we have been stressed. And it is estimated that most of the health complaints patients tell the doctor, are highly associated with stress. It is, therefore, critical to avoid or to a large extent reduce on what stresses us, because this may have an adverse and negative effect on our health.

LAST WORDS

Health is indeed a critical choice and it is highly individualised. As someone who minds his or her health, keep in mind and accentuate that nearly all non-communicable, chronic diseases can be preventable and reversible through the dedicated choices you could make on nutrition and lifestyle.

The notion that some diseases *"run in our family"* should not be used as a premise to relax and let things be. Some people do not do anything about their deteriorating health because *"that's how my father and mother are or were, as well, it's in our genes."* Wrong! The genes can be altered in the way they express and your current environment plays a bigger role. Genes should not determine your health or life destiny because, true to it, *genes can load the gun, but it is the environment that pulls the trigger.*

As human beings, we need to have a holistic approach to our health in order to be in optimal conditions. This means we need to address our physical, emotional and even spiritual wellbeing. Studies show that people with a high inclination to believing in something higher or superior being, (God, for example), rate higher in terms of health, albeit not forgetting that they do eat aptly and not be a *couch potato.*

Just because you think you feel fine right now, despite eating highly processed foods and leading a sedentary life, does not mean all is well. Chronic illness takes time to come out. Act now! Do not get fixated at the idea that getting sick is normal and the doctor is there to heal you. Instead prescribe your own medicine, as Hippocrates said, *"Let food be thy medicine and medicine be thy food."*

THANK YOUS!

Writing books is tougher than I imagined and more fulfilling than I could have ever envisioned. Having an idea and turning into a book, is not an easy thing at all. The activity is both intrinsically rough but worthwhile. None of this would have been feasible devoid of moral support from you my precious family. You stood by my side during those late hours and endless printing and shredding of paper and what not, during the writing of this valuable book. That is real love.

Scribbling a book about health and nutrition is a colossal task because information about the subject changes every minute and it remains a subject that keeps on having diverse and opposing views. I am forever indebted to my editorial team for the keen acumen and constant support in bringing this book to fruition. It is because of their hard work and reassurance that I have the legacy to have this book out for people to learn and appreciate health and wellness.

To all of you my friends who contributed in one way or another, know that the world is a much better place thanks to individuals like yourselves who want to see a better, healthier and happier world through food and lifestyle changes in life. That is true friendship.

AJB

REFERENCES

Brukner Peter, 2018, *A Fat Lot Of Good*, Penguin Random House Australia.

Campbell T. Collin, Campbell Thomas M, 2016, *The China Study*, Ben Bella Books Inc. Dallas Texas.

Carr Kris, 2011, *Crazy Sexy Diet*, Skirt, an imprint of Globe Pequot Press, USA.

Francis Raymond, 2002, *Never Be Sick Again*, Health Communications inc, Deerfield Beach, Florida.

Francis Raymond, 2014, *The Great American Health Hoax*, Health Communications inc, Deerfield Beach, Florida.

Fuhrman Joel, 2011, *Super Immunity*, Harper One, an Imprint of Harper Collins Publishers, New York.

Greger Michael, 2015, *How Not To Die*, Pan Books, an imprint of Pan Macmillan, UK.

Lustig Robert, 2013, *Fat Chance*, Fourth Estate, Harper Collins Publishers, London.

Pollan Michael, 2008, *In Defence of Food, an Eater's Manifesto*, Penguin Group, USA.

William Anthony, 2015, *Medical Medium*, Hay House, printed in Australia by McPherson's Printing Group.

Yudkin John, 1972, 1986, *Pure, White and Deadly*, Penguin Life, UK, an Imprint of Penguin Books.